THE MUSIC CAME FROM DEEP INSIDE

One day I went into Eileen's room and after we did the "band sound" activity, she said, "You know, Reggie can sing. He's learned 'Comin' Round the Mountain.'" Reggie's a large, profoundly retarded black boy of 18. Well—I started that song and then I stopped, and Eileen said, "C'mon, Reggie, it's your turn." And it was like that music came from way far inside of him, but he worked at it and worked at it and finally did it twice all the way through—kind of husky and soft. It was wonderful—and I'm going to get him to learn some more of those folk songs.

Michele Valeri (Music)
Great Oaks Arts Team

The contribution you, as artists, are making here is partly this: because of what you *are* and what you are able to give of yourself, you have a unique capacity to block out all the visible trappings of what these children are and reach deep into the human being trapped inside.

You've selected your own art form because of what *you* are. And you're going to use it to see if, somehow, we can turn this human situation around . . . to inch it on to whatever percentage *more* it can be! What it might really *become*, for any given child who rides out there on your artistry, is just awesome!

George Latshaw (Puppeteer)
and principal project artist)
to the Walton Arts Team

THE MUSIC CAME FROM DEEP INSIDE

A Story of Artists and Severely Handicapped Children

JUNIUS EDDY

Photographs by Roger Vaughan
Introduction by
ROBERT COLES, M.D.

McGRAW-HILL BOOK COMPANY
New York   St. Louis   San Francisco
London   Paris   Singapore   Tokyo   Toronto

Thomas H. Quinn and Michael Hennelly were the editors
of this book. Elaine Gongora was the designer. Sally Fliess
supervised the production. It was set in Century
Schoolbook by Allyn-Mason, Inc.

Printed and bound by R. R. Donnelley and Sons, Inc.

This book is an account of a project administered by the
National Committee/Arts for the Handicapped. The project
was partially supported by a grant from the Bureau of
Education for the Handicapped, Division of Innovation and
Development, U.S. Office of Education, Washington, D.C.

Library of Congress Cataloging in Publication Data
Eddy, Junius.
    The music came from deep inside.

    1. Mentally handicapped children—Education—United
States—Arts—Case studies. I. Title.
LC4025.E33   371.92′83   82-15192
                                       AACR2

ISBN 0-07-018971-4

1 2 3 4 5 6 7 8 9 DO DO 8 9 8 7 6 5 4 3 2

CONTENTS

ON RENEWING
TEACHER CREATIVITY

We're doing something terribly important for the humanization of these teachers . . . renewing their creativity maybe. They're so damned proud of their kids—and it seems to me that what's going on in these projects may have a real impact on the tendency teachers have, in this business, to feel trapped, unable to go farther, burned-out. Here, though (perhaps in these festivals especially), they can see what their kids are getting out of it and it may help them get more involved in this whole arts approach.

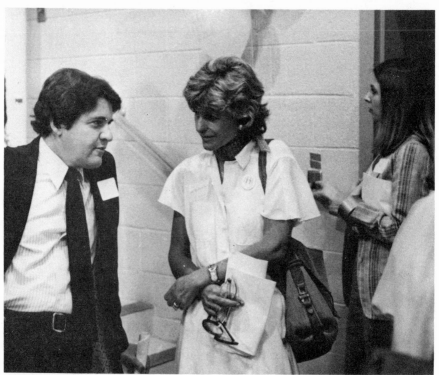

NCAH Founder Jean Kennedy Smith with Edwin Martin, former Director of USOE's Bureau of Education For the Handicapped, at the Great Oaks Very Special Arts Festival.

One of the great and serious problems in work of this kind is how do you keep people working with continuing satisfaction in a place like this, how do you give them reinforcement, how do you keep them from getting to feel *un*creative, *un*productive and ultimately depressed?

To see these dedicated and committed teachers doing things like this with their kids—well, it's a lesson, really—because it's the things you do yourself that often teach you the most and so, when they do these things in the arts, they *learn* it. And as they're doing it, they're proving the humanness of these kids all over again, to themselves.

Edwin W. Martin
Former Deputy Commissioner of Education and
Director, Bureau of Education For the Handicapped, U.S. Office of Education

PREFACE

THIS NARRATIVE is an account of a journey that Roger Vaughan and I made recently into a world that the vast majority of Americans knows little about and does not willingly enter. It is a world in which demons are sometimes thought to lurk; a world where humanity is occasionally hidden deep inside an inanimate appearance, where the traditional road maps are of little use to those unfamiliar with the terrain, and where (among other attributes) extraordinary care and patience are demanded of those who work there.

Yet once we entered it and, so to speak, our eyes became accustomed to the darkness, we found it a world of infinite wonder and—frequently—delight.

For this world is inhabited by children. Exceptional children. Special children. Special because they are, in fact, among the incomprehensible exceptions to the human scheme of things—a terrible ironic joke on mankind. For these children function at what are termed the severe and profound levels of mental retardation and handicap. Whatever their chronological age, by most developmental criteria only a very few of these children will ever progress beyond this world of early childhood.

They are what Wendy Perks, former executive director of the National Committee, Arts for the Handicapped, called "the last of the least." She has said, "They are the least capable of taking care of themselves. They have received the least attention. They are the toughest kids to reach. They don't make good poster children."

It is estimated that some 460,000 children and youth between the ages of birth and 19 live in this twilight world. In the course of our journey, Roger Vaughan and I became acquainted with perhaps 300 of these children; of that number we ultimately became rather deeply involved in the lives of about two dozen. Many of them, we like to think, came to be our friends.

We found these children, and the adults who teach and care for them, in three small, somewhat dissimilar school environments in Texas, California, and Maryland. The schools had been selected by members of the Washington-based staff of the National Committee, Arts for the Handicapped, to serve as the sites for an unusually challenging three-year project. We had been asked to document, in words and photographs, what occurred during the project's first operational year.

Designed to bring the unique talents of professional artists to bear on the lives and learning tasks of these 300 children, the project began with an orientation meeting for site personnel, documenters, and evaluators in Washington in November 1978. The pilot year ended with a series of exuberant celebrations—called Very Special Arts Festivals by the National Committee—at each project site during the early summer of 1979.

Our assignment was focused, of course, on what happened in between, as the intervention process took place. And for this, we simply went along—on a number of occasions—when George Latshaw, a professional puppeteer, and three separate teams of artists were exploring new ways of reaching, motivating, and teaching these children who occupy the lowest rung of the developmental ladder.

This book represents the formal outcomes of that assignment. But it is something considerably more than that for us. In putting it together, we have been more conscious perhaps than ever before in our professional lives of our responsibility to our subjects. It's essential that we keep faith with those children, with their teachers, and with the artists whose creative energies were focused on them both during this period. If we have managed to portray accurately the range and richness of personality, and the true nature of the artistry that made the whole experience memorable, then we will have found the best way possible to give back something in return for the privilege of being there with them, for a time.

I verge on sentimentality here—and that is one of the pitfalls when one attempts to write about these children. Neither Vaughan nor I had any previous experience with children like these—certainly not in groups this large. Furthermore, neither of us knew very much about the field of special education, at *any* level of retardation and handicap. Working on this project was like a plunge into an icy steam for us. It has been difficult, in consequence, to avoid a kind of heart-on-your-sleeve reaction when it comes to reporting about such painful and touching circumstances as these.

But, bearing this in mind, we have tried to cultivate, in our reporting, that admirable blend of fondness and tough-mindedness we found in almost all the best teachers of these children. Perhaps some of the gifted unconventionality of the artists has rubbed off on us too—and given us some necessary new insights into the human condition.

Here then—in my words and Roger Vaughan's pictures—is the story of the first year of this project as we saw it during our journey into the world of these badly damaged children.

Junius Eddy
Little Compton, R.I.

INTRODUCTION
Robert Coles

WHEN I WORKED in the rural South and in Appalachia I sometimes met children such as this book describes—children I was quick to designate as "retarded," as "severely handicapped." I took note of "behavior." I was told about a given "school performance." I heard from a doctor or a teacher about one or another kind of "emotional disorder." But the families I met, often enough, were not inclined to such ways of putting things. Here is how I heard one youth of fourteen talk about her seven-year-old brother: "He was sent to us by God, and He decided that Jimmie should be slow, and take life easier than most of us. You know, the soul is not the mind. You know, it's not through the smarts that you get into God's favor, and He takes you into Heaven. You know, our minister keeps telling us that God is Love, and my momma says 'amen, amen' when we hear the minister say so, and when we look at our brother, and he's in trouble, and he can't do this, and he can't do that, and we start snickering, my mother calls us over, and she reminds us of what we've heard in church, and she tells us that our brother is a gift of God's. We all are, and we're here because He wanted us to be here, and if we don't know that about one of us, we don't know it about ourselves, or our best friends, or anyone. So we'd better stop and think and not be so sure *we're* the biggest, most important persons in the whole, wide world!"

A youth with no great educational "background," with no great promise as a scholar or researcher. A youth who, as a matter of fact, was all too readily regarded by me as "culturally disadvantaged" talking about the ways we put down, dismiss, arrogantly categorize others, thereby demeaning and revealing all too dismally our own selves! Yet, a youth who saw what an itinerant Gallilean teacher and healer along ago meant, as He kept company so insistently with the lame, the halt, the blind, the rebuked and the scorned, the hurt and the troubled.

In the book that follows we are reminded that hope is everywhere, no matter the apparent lack of promise in a particular person or group of people. We are reminded that no one is beyond our ken—our touch, our interest, our disciplined, knowing resolve. The "problem" is not only "them," the children who are "severely and profoundly handicapped." The "problem" is, as always, ourselves—our assumptions, our blindspots, our prejudices and unyielding preferences, and yes, our terrible pride. Junius Eddy and Roger Vaughan bring us close, indeed, to these quite special children—but also, quite close to ourselves, and the difficulties in us that often stand in the way of the service we might offer to others. That child quoted above knew how often self-centredness, self-regard keep us from seeing the possibilities in others. I'm not so sure that many of us who have no so-called "handicaps" of the conventional kind don't, in fact, suffer from the greatest handicap of all—the prideful sense that only *we* are truly human and significant, we whose minds have a certain "I.Q.," a certain "education," a certain "training."

The words that follow, the photographs, too, amount in their sum to a measure of possible hope—for the reader, for the person who will work with the handicapped, as well as for "them," those thousands and thousands of boys and girls who are here among us, fellow creatures, travellers like us on this uncertain voyage called "life," and not least, potential teachers themselves, in the sense that they can reveal to us much about our aspirations, our limitations. "Grace is everywhere," wrote the French novelist Bernanos in his great novel *The Diary of a Country Priest*, and we are all possible instruments of that grace—certainly including the boys and girls whose stories, whose appearance we encounter in this book. Nor, in that regard, should the book itself be denied its providential character—words and images of dedicated, thoughtful concern, of continuing and loving attentiveness, sent our lucky way.

THE PROJECT

IT IS UNLIKELY that a project focused on such a discrete population as the severely and profoundly handicapped could have emerged much earlier in the recent, and brief, history of arts education in the United States. This project, whose full official title is "A Model Program of Arts to Enhance Living and Learning for Severely and Profoundly Handicapped Children and Youth", is unique, a first of its kind for the National Committee, Arts for the Handicapped (NCAH), and also for the various partners to the enterprise. A lot of programmatic underbrush had to be cleared out of the way first. The idea had to grow organically through a series of developmental stages in the arts education field—first in general education and then in special education—until finally there was nobody left unserved but those Wendy Perks, the first NCAH executive director, has called "the last of the least."

Of course, when it comes to reaping the benefits of public and private support for arts education, the handicapped population generally has been pretty well ignored (as it had been in many other areas of social endeavor, some of its advocates would say). Certainly, in so far as federal attention and federal dollars are concerned, the handicapped were the last to be invited to the arts education table—not until 1975, the year the National Committee was established. This also was the year that Public Law 94-142, the landmark handicapped education act, was signed into law.

To be sure, that arts education table had only been visibly set since the mid-1960s and, for most of that

Public Law 94-142

Public Law 94-142 is the popular term for the Education for All Handicapped Children Act, the landmark legislation that Congress passed in 1975 in the special education field, which has significant implications for severely and profoundly handicapped youngsters in particular.

Public Law 94-142 requires that every state and local school district receiving federal funds must find and educate *at public expense* all handicapped children in its jurisdiction, regardless of the nature and severity of a child's handicap.

It also called for states to start educating handicapped children of pre-school age by September of 1978 and handicapped youths aged 18 to 21 by September of 1980, *if* education for *nonhandicapped* students in these age ranges was also regularly provided.

For the estimated 3.6 million handicapped children between 6 and 17 years of age, the law specifies that school districts shall:

Make every reasonable effort to locate handicapped children and give first priority to the most severely disabled. Thus, the law's most dramatic effect has been the so-called Child-Find Program, aimed at locating children in those SPH (severely and profoundly handicapped) categories either in institutions or at home who were receiving no education but

time, it's been placed off in a corner somewhere away from the main festive board the government has prepared for the educational powers that be. The table has never been particularly overflowing, either. For the last 15 years, in fact, the serving at that table might best be described as a child's portion. A portion that had to be divided still further when the handicapped drew up a chair.

Nonetheless, meager as the Federal sustenance may have been, it did manage to stimulate some early arts education action, under the Elementary and Secondary Education Act of 1965. ESEA's Title I (compensatory education for the disadvantaged) and who are now entitled to be educated at public expense. The cost of educating such children has also shifted from parents and other public agencies to the school systems.

Evaluate the learning needs of each child, in consultation with parents and special education advisors, and develop an individual education program to meet these needs. Much of the burden for developing these "IEPs" (individual education plans) has fallen on homeroom teachers but, although compliance is said to be mixed, the vast majority of handicapped children seem now to have had such programs prescribed.

Place each child in the least restricted environment possi- *ble, whether this be a hospital, a state institution, a private day school, a public school special education program, or a regular classroom.* This is the so-called mainstreaming provision. It allows institutionalized children to be transferred to special classes in regular public schools. Furthermore, it provides that children who were formerly in special classes in the public schools *may* spend part of their time "mainstreamed" in regular classes.

Periodically evaluate the child's progress and make changes in the IEP if needed, again with parents and specialists participating in these changes.

Title III (educational innovation) were especially notable for the number of pioneering school-based projects in the arts that were launched in the late 1960s. By the early seventies the National Endowment for the Arts began, somewhat cautiously, to enter the education arena by establishing what has now become its major activity in this field, the Artists-in-Schools Program (recently renamed Artists in Education Program).

Meanwhile, back in the private sector, similar but generally separate activities concerned with arts education began to receive support from the foundation world at critical points during that decade. And ultimately, out of this period of innovation and ferment, there emerged a kind of national movement, a groundswell of conviction among educators and artists alike, about the critical importance of the arts to many aspects of the educational process.

As one finds this conviction expressed in various school programs around the country, they appear to be based on two rather fundamental assumptions. The first is that the arts have educational value in and of themselves because they add significantly to the quality of one's life and contribute to the development of the whole person, the fully functioning individual. And the second is that the arts have a utilitarian value in education because they are a powerful (if long neglected) teaching and learning tool, something teachers can use everyday in their classrooms to generate learnings in other academic areas and to nurture aspects of the children's social and personal growth. Moreover, there is beginning to be a substantial body of research to back up these assumptions.

But what about the child who is *not* fully functioning, who will never be a whole person in one or more very crucial ways? Can the arts enhance the quality of that life? Can the arts indeed be used to reach, motivate, and teach such a child?

These were questions only a handful of special education people were even asking 15 years ago. There were few clues being unearthed that might have helped to answer them, either, other than the insights provided by some imaginative arts therapists, a few educational psychologists and philosophers, and the perceptive teachers of so-called learning-disability children. And these questions remained largely unanswered until 1974 when the entire issue was given visibility at a national conference supported by the Joseph P. Kennedy, Jr., Foundation and organized to explore the role of the arts in meeting the needs of the mentally retarded.

It was out of this conference, and several others that followed, that the National Committee, Arts for the Handicapped, emerged on the national scene in 1975, with a lively mandate to "do something" but practically no funds to do it with. It found a tentative "home" at the Kennedy Center for the Performing Arts, however, under the protective wing of the Alliance for Arts Education (AAE). The AAE is the Kennedy Center's educational arm and had itself been established in 1973 as a joint effort of the Center and the U.S. Office of Education.

Then, in 1976, the federal reserve began to crack. Congress provided $1 million to support the programs of the Alliance—and that amount included $250,000 earmarked specifically for the work of the National Committee. In 1977 this was increased to $500,000, in 1978 to $1 million, and in 1979 to $1.5 million where it now stands.

In the half-dozen years of its existence, the NCAH has managed to secure grants from the Office (now Department) of Education and other sources, public and private, to augment the funds it gets directly from Congress each year. The combined annual budget is certainly not munificent, but it has enabled the hardworking NCAH staff (still allied with the AAE but now working out of a small, bustling office in downtown Washington) to put some of its dreams into operation.

By 1978–79, under Wendy Perks's energetic leadership, "arts for the handicapped" projects or activities were in place at more than eighty different sites around the nation—and their number has grown steadily since. Many, naturally, were in school settings; some were established to develop model demonstration programs; others were set up as regional resource and information centers; still others enabled professionals in the field to develop teaching guides and undertake needed research and dissemination efforts. NCAH has also organized numerous

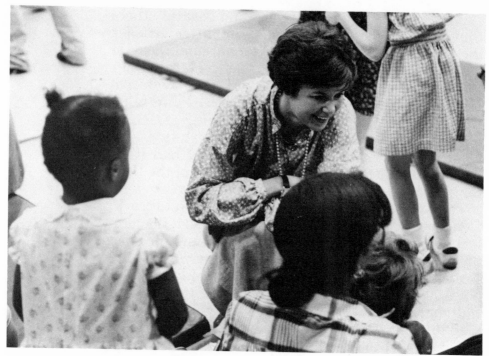

Wendy Perks and Great Oaks children.

regional training sessions to prepare a cadre of state
and local leaders who could stage the Very Special
Arts Festivals, events aimed at raising a community's consciousness as well as celebrating the lives
and learnings of its exceptional children.

Until 1978, however, only one of these arts projects
was designed specifically to reach these most damaged and vulnerable of children—the severely and
profoundly handicapped. The single exception was a
month-long pilot project in the spring of that year
which brought puppeteer George Latshaw to the
Great Oaks Center in Maryland for a month-long
involvement with fifteen of these children and their
teachers.

So convincing were the results of this pilot that
NCAH administrators—and then Associate Director
Louise Appell in particular—believed that a greatly

expanded effort should be made to explore what the arts might accomplish with this population.

Dr. Appell had come to the National Committee in 1976 from Catholic University in Washington where she was director of the graduate program in special education. Whether as teacher, administrator, or researcher, she had immersed herself in the world of handicapped children for most of her adult life. And, because they present the greatest challenge, children with severe and profound handicapping conditions had become of particular concern to her in recent years.

So Louise Appell and Wendy Perks set to work on a proposal designed specifically for this population. They planned to base their proposal on an already existing arts program NCAH had developed as a model for working with the mildly and moderately handicapped; the concept would be refined and then adapted to meet the special needs of children and youth in the severe/profound category. They saw it as a 3-year venture, in which the first year would be perhaps the most critical one because it would be devoted to shaping and developing the new model in three quite diverse pilot sites. During the project's second and third years NCAH would replicate the program in perhaps a dozen new sites, field test it, and produce an arts activities manual and a how-to-do-it guide for implementing the model in still other settings which served severe and profound populations. (See "Afterword" for details on years 2 and 3).

There were two intertwined project goals: one proposed to improve *the quality of life* for severely and profoundly handicapped children and youth through a variety of experiences in the arts; the other proposed to improve *the functional skills* of these children through the use of arts strategies—clearly the more challenging aim of the two. The art forms to be introduced at each project site were puppetry (in the person of George Latshaw), music, the visual arts, dance, and drama. A team comprised of professional artists representing the latter four major art forms was to be engaged in each locality.

It added up to a bold and ambitious program—and a costly one. But Perks and Appell planned to submit their proposal to the U.S. Office of Education's Bureau of Education for the Handicapped (BEH) which, just a year earlier, had been authorized to provide funding for what were termed "model programs"; twenty-four model projects had been supported the first year, but none had dealt in any way with the arts. Furthermore, the BEH* had recently established as a priority objective the development of educational projects for children in the severe and profound categories which would enable such children "to become as independent as possible, thereby reducing their requirements for institutional care, and providing opportunities for self-development." To Perks's and Appell's way of thinking, their NCAH proposal was directly on target in both instances.

And indeed it must have been, because BEH ultimately did approve the project for first-year funding and indicated it would look favorably on second and third year continuation requests.

Now the project so close to Perks's and Appell's hearts could proceed. Finally the opportunity was at hand to enlist the unique contributions of the arts on behalf of these special kids—in a systematic attempt to prove what Louise Appell believed so passionately; namely, that "no level of human activity is so deficient as to preclude learning" and that "the arts can become a valuable learning tool even at this extreme of the developmental continuum."

A delay in receiving the funds meant that the project could not begin, as intended, with the opening of the 1978 school year. However, by November, the funds were in place and some critical decisions had

*In May of 1980, BEH became the Office of Special Education in the newly created Education Department.

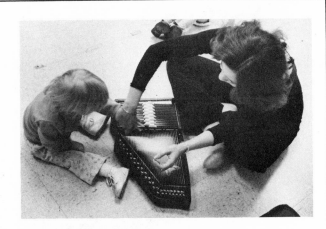

The Arts
and
Handicapped Children

. . . it is well to start thinking of using the arts especially when you want to introduce an approach that is nonthreatening to a vulnerable child, or to teach a basic skill in a new way, or to stimulate your student's creativity.

. . . The potential the arts have for enriching the life experiences of handicapped children, for improving the self-image, for stimulating the senses, and for motivating the reluctant and recalcitrant are best realized when they are presented systematically, routinely, and repeatedly. The first successful performance is rewarding, the second and third are reassuring, but the fourth is convincing.

There is an excitement about teaching and learning through the arts that is evident to any observer who might stop by your classroom.

Exuberance, eagerness, and delight are usual. Some children will surprise you. The lethargic and withdrawn child will become animated; the undisciplined and easily distracted child may become focused; and the angry and disruptive child may become docile and helpful.

It is important to be open and flexible, to be willing to try something a little different, and to shed some stereotypes. Most of all it is important to enjoy!

"Arts for Learning" Teacher's Guide
(developed under an NCAH grant)

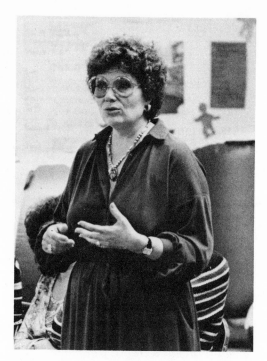

Louise Appell at Walton orientation session.

been made: the three sites had been chosen (after a number of possible facilities has been visited by Appell during the selection process); NCAH staffer Ralph Nappi, who had coordinated an earlier pilot at Great Oaks, had been named project coordinator; puppeteer George Latshaw's experience in the pilot made him the *only* possible choice as principal artist; Dr. Hugh Mcbride, an educational psychologist in the School of Education at University of the Pacific in Stockton, California, had been asked to take on the role of project evaluator/data analyst; and Roger Vaughan and I had agreed to undertake the documentation tasks, in words and pictures.

In addition, an administrative team had been appointed for each site consisting of an administrative director and a site team leader; the latter's job was to work in close cooperation with the pilot school and to coordinate the activities of the team of artists selected to work in the classrooms—with Latshaw's periodic visits working as a catalytic influence to weld these various artist-teacher relationships into productive alliances.

All parties to the enterprise (except the three teams of artists) came to Washington in November to attend an orientation session conducted by the Perks-Appell Administrative Team at NCAH. At that meeting, Vaughan and I met the administrative teams from each project site for the first time and learned something about the three schools we'd be visiting frequently during the course of the next six months.

THE PILOT SITES

THE PILOT SCHOOL settings, their administrative structures, and the amount of parent involvement differed considerably, we found, from site to site. These distinctions were not accidental. They were built into the selection criteria by NCAH in order to represent as much of the institutional diversity within the special education field as possible—and particularly in those facilities serving severely and profoundly handicapped children.

It may be well, at this point, to make clear some of those distinctions—as of 1978–79 when the project began.

The Great Oaks Center

One of the sites almost selected itself. This was the Great Oaks Center, a large residental facility tucked away in the hills of Maryland a few miles north of Silver Spring. For one thing, it had been the scene of Latshaw's month-long pilot the previous spring and there was a built-in readiness among the staff to explore the arts process further. For another, it is only a 45-minute drive from the District of Columbia and could serve as a kind of "show-and-tell" site where BEH, NCAH, and other Washington folk could drop in occasionally and see what was going on. But probably most important, Great Oaks is the first *regional* residential center to be planned and operated by the state of Maryland—it opened in 1970—and as such it coordinates a continuum of services for the mentally retarded and their families in five Maryland counties.

Great Oaks, we learned, is by far the most complex of the three institutions serving as project sites. It operates as a unit of the Mental Retardation Administration within the state's Department of Health and Mental Hygiene. The center's facilities consist of a mazelike arrangement of dormitories, special care wards, dining areas, classrooms, and administrative buildings that spread across the grounds and are, for the most part, connected by covered walkways. The school building proper sits on a hill that overlooks the rest of the complex.

Presently some 470 mentally retarded children and adults live at the center, those requiring constant care in the dormitories, and those who are less dependent in cottages apart from the main complex. Most are classed, developmentally, in the severe and profound levels of retardation. Many have one or more physical handicaps as well.

About half the Great Oaks residents are under 21 and, in Maryland, therefore, of school age. Of this group, about half have already been affected by Public Law 94-192 and are attending the public schools in neighboring communities. This group consists almost entirely of children who have been diagnosed as "mildly" or "moderately" handicapped for whom the public schools are a "less restrictive environment" than the Great Oaks School. The other half—nearly 110 young children and adolescents—go to school at the center; about 90 to 95 percent of them are severely and profoundly retarded. They were our "project children."

Each weekday morning, with the assistance of a lively corps of "foster grandparents," these children are loaded into buses at their living quarters on the center grounds. They are driven the short distance up the hill to the two-story Great Oaks School where their teachers and teacher aides are gathered to meet them as they come off the buses. The "walkers" enter at the upper level and those in wheelchairs are brought to the lower level. (One of my earliest im-

The Foster Grandparent Program

Great Oaks staffers believe that the Foster Grandparent Program has played a central role in creating a new sense of family for many of the children. This is a long-term, federally supported program under which elderly people in the community are engaged (on a modest monthly stipend) to minister to some of the needs of children who cannot care for themselves. They must be senior citizens with low incomes to qualify as foster grandparents.

At Great Oaks the "grannies", as the school staff calls them, include four foster grandfathers in what is otherwise pretty much a maternal group. They are bused in from their homes in Prince Georges County to spend 4 hours a day with the children who've been assigned to them, generally those confined to a wheelchair existence. They come, a dozen or so strong, on each of two shifts (morning and afternoon) designed to span the school day and thereby help the hard-pressed teaching staff with basic-care tasks.

The remarks (opposite page) of Mrs. Laura Caldwell, a warm and active woman in her 80s who has been the foster grandmother of an 11-year-old boy named Billy for seven years, are typical of how these men and women feel about their tasks and their "children".

pressions of Great Oaks is the loudspeaker announcement that alerts the teachers each morning: "The ambulatory bus is now arriving at the upper level" and "The nonambulatory bus is now arriving at the lower level").

Here, for the next 6 hours, the special education of these special children takes place—in the dozen or more colorful and uniquely equipped classrooms and the halls and ramps leading to them. There are

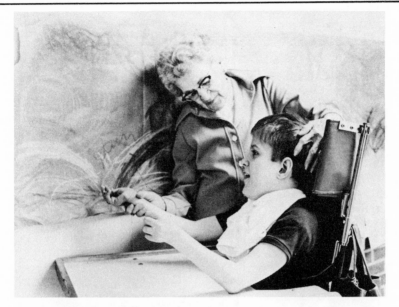

Mrs. Caldwell and Billy. (Photo by Molly A. Roberts)

For a couple of years after my husband died, I struggled along pretty much alone. Then one day I saw in the paper about this sort of work—with cerebral palsy children—and when they took me up there and I saw all those children in wheelchairs, crawling on the floor, or using crutches, I thought "why am I feeling sorry for myself? They need me and I need them." The fact is I really needed them more than they needed me.

I got Billy [diagnosed as a spastic quadraplegic] when he was 4 years old. From what I understand, Billy is a "state child." They took me up to Billy's bed in the unit and when he looked up at me and smiled, I was gone. Billy's my child—I knew it right then. Even now, when I'm feeling down and out, I can look at him and see that smile and it does me so much good!

If I was younger and had the money, Billy wouldn't be here. I'm working with lovely people, of course, the teachers and all—and I must say that since I've been helping with Billy and these other children, I feel God has given me something special. I used to say "God, please help me make somebody happy" and so far I think—at least I hope—I'm making some of these children happy.

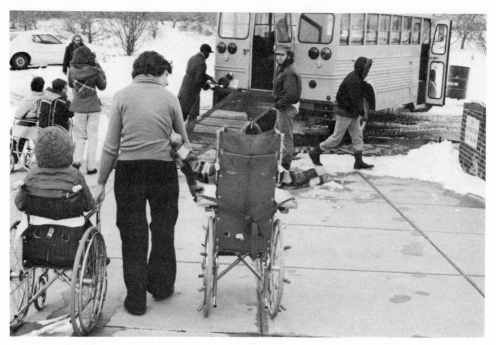

Loading the "non-ambulatory bus" after school at Great Oaks.

about twenty-one certified special education teachers and perhaps fifteen teacher aides assigned to the
Great Oaks classrooms, a ratio of about one adult for
each three children. Except for special activities or
events, there are generally no more than six or
seven children in any classroom, and sometimes
only three or four if they require constant care.

When the school day ends, at 3:00 in the afternoon, the buses pull up outside once again, and the
teachers, the aides, and the foster grandparents
bring the children out on the ramps and assist the
bus crew with the loading process. Some of the walkers lend a hand with their less coordinated but still
ambulatory classmates. And then the buses drive
back down the hill again and deliver the children to
their living quaters, where the dormitory staff

provides the care they need during the nonschool part of their lives.

The in-school part is administered by a principal, Stuart Poltilove; assistant principal, Judy Wierenga; and two education supervisors, Jeanne Holsey and Lynn Johnson. One of the supervisors, Lynn Johnson, was selected by Poltilove, the Great Oaks liaison to NCAH, to serve as the project's administrative director there. Janet Goodrich, whose career has included acting, directing, and producing for the professional theater, was picked to be the site team leader and coordinate the artists' intervention tasks.

To be "institutionalized" as a mentally retarded or handicapped person is, at Great Oaks, a far cry from the traditional snake-pit implications of that term. Indeed, it may be one of the most enlightened institutions of its kind anywhere. Still, the children who are placed there no longer belong to a family, in the true sense. Some, of course, have either been abandoned or have no living relatives and are, therefore, wards of the state; others have been placed here by their parents and, like Blanche Dubois in the Tennessee Williams play, must now depend on the kindness of strangers.

At Great Oaks, however, as parental visits get farther and farther apart and often cease altogether, the strangers soon become familiar of face, voice, and touch. Before long it is the dormitory staff, the teachers, and the foster grandparents (see box) who have become the child's true family.

The Special Care School

The other two project facilities are in rather striking contrast to the institutional ambiance of the Great Oaks Center, if not to the hilltop school itself. You approach the other two schools through streets that crisscross what are essentially middle-class suburban developments—and there, as you turn a corner, is what appears to be the neighborhood elementary

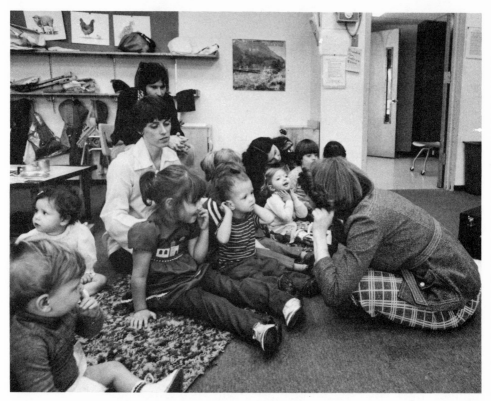

Children and teachers in a Special Care School classroom.

school, smaller than most but typical of today's one-story, flat-roof brick construction.

In Texas, it is the Special Care School, located in northwest Dallas County on 3½ acres of land in a district known as Farmers Branch. In California, it is the Roger Walton Development Center situated on public school acreage next to Stagg High School on the northwest edge of Stockton, where the Calaveras River runs between the school and the campus of the University of the Pacific, just to the south.

The Special Care School (SCS) is a private, non-profit day school for children 3 to 21 years of age who are mentally retarded, brain damaged, or are physically and emotionally handicapped. Some trainable adolescents and adults are taught in a "sheltered workshop" situation in the Task Training Center, and Extended Day Care (from 7 A.M. to 6 P.M.) is offered to young handicapped children of working parents.

The school was founded under church sponsorship in the mid-1960s. It is supported variously by contributions, small grants from local businesses and civic organizations, and by the United Way program in the Dallas area. But its main sources of support since it opened its new brick facility in 1971 have been the contracts it receives from nearby school systems, and mainly the Dallas Independent School District.

These contracts, in effect, purchase from the Special Care School the so-called appropriate education which the school systems themselves have not heretofore been able to provide for their district's most severely disabled students. Earlier, SCS served mildly and moderately retarded students as well, but gradually children in these categories have been shifted back to regular school settings as the districts began implementing Public Law 94-192 (as well as the pioneering Texas legislation, SB 230, which was passed in 1970 and, Texans assert, was really the model for the 1975 federal law).

Carol Fritze, the dynamic director of the Special Care School, says that this situation means some serious readjustments for SCS in the very near future. "More and more," she points out, "districts are saying they can take these kids and provide an appropriate education for them—so they no longer need the contracts with us. But parents who've been operating on contracts for up to 10 years are often quite upset at the prospect of their child going to public school. Sometimes their concerns are justified and sometimes they're not."

Parents can either keep their child at SCS and pay the tuition costs, or they can ask the school to appeal

Special Care School: Program Description

The Special Care School provides a program appropriate to the needs of each individual student, planned by the school staff in conjunction with the student's family. Depending on his needs, the student is placed in one of the following classes:

Multiage Training Class— emphasizes basic self-care needs of sitting, walking, eating, toileting, attending to task, and basic communications relating to self-care.

Infant Stimulation Class (mornings only)—children from birth to 3 years of age; emphasis on sensory motor and fine motor skills, language development, toileting, and eating.

*Primary Class—*young children needing an emphasis on self-care skills of eating, toileting, and gross motor development, attending skills, language development, play, and socialization.

*Transitional Class—*young students who have mastered vital self-care skills; increased emphasis on language development, play and socialization skills, prevocational skills, and preacademic/academic skills.

the district's decision. In several instances recently, SCS has won such appeals. But the trend appears to be unmistakable and, as more and more school districts respond to the mandates of Public Law 94-192 and attempt to make provision for an "appropriate education" for youngsters lower and lower on the developmental ladder, schools like SCS must look for alternatives.

"One of the things we're looking at here," says Carol Fritze, "is enlarging our Day Care Program considerably. We're trying to work out arrangements with the Department of Human Re-

Intermediate I—adolescent and adult students needing an emphasis on academic skills, home living, prevocational and vocational skills, advanced self-care, and leisure time.

Intermediate II—adolescent and adult students needing an emphasis on functional language, advanced self-care, prevocational and home living skills, and leisure time.

Behavior-Management Class—multiage grouping of students who can profit from a highly structured program to increase attending skills, toileting skills, modeling behaviors, and appropriate language skills.

During the life of the project at SCS, the Multiage Training Class contained six children designated as "profoundly retarded" and both the Intermediate II Class (with eight to nine children) and the Behavior-Management Class (with six children) were designated as "severely retarded." The rest of the children were said to be either too young to be accurately diagnosed or older and verging on the TMR category: trainable mentally retarded.

sources to have a day-care setup for relatively normal kids. It would give us a chance to mix the mentally retarded kids already in our day-care program with the higher-level kids—and that would provide stimulation for our kids and help the others learn some compassion for the handicapped."

At present, however, there are nearly sixty students attending SCS—and most are still on school district contracts. Some parents drive their children to and from school each day; the rest are transported by school buses with special lifts for wheelchair riders. The children range from the older, so-called

trainable youngsters to the very young—those up to
3 years of age, including some under 18 months who
are what the school refers to as "developmentally delayed" children. This is a term (another is "language
delayed") coming into increasing use in order not to
label as "mentally retarded" very young children
who may simply develop normal actions and behaviors *later* than other children. Many, in fact, are
just too young to be diagnosed yet.

There are seven sunny, pleasant, and visually
stimulating classrooms at SCS, each under the professional supervision of a certified "special ed"
teacher with the assistance of one or more paraprofessionals. Practicum students and volunteers frequently help out in the classrooms as well. The staff
also includes three therapists (physical, occupa-
tional, and speech/language) and a part-time recreation specialist. In addition to its classrooms, the
school has outdoor play courts, a good-sized gymnasium, a special "task training room," and a room
set aside for "art—music—talk—sign language."

There is a developmental sequence to the various
classrooms, and their descriptions (see box) tell a
good deal about the diverse and complicated world of
handicapped and retarded children.

Many of the practicum students who come in and
out of the Special Care School are enrolled at Texas
Woman's University (TWU) in Denton, 25 miles to
the north. Among other distinctions, TWU has
developed a special competency in the field of
"adapted physical education and recreation," due
almost entirely to the pioneering work of Dr.
Claudine Sherrill, who has held a full professorship
there since 1971. Dr. Sherrill teaches at TWU's College of Health, Physical Education and Recreation
and her graduate courses, which are focused sharply
on the role of the arts—and dance especially—in
therapeutic work with the handicapped, are widely
recognized and highly regarded throughout the
country.

She has also directed several Bureau of Education for the Handicapped (BEH)-funded projects in recent years, one of which—an Inservice Education Project in Creative Arts for the Handicapped—was still going on when the NCAH project began. These factors, plus her wide-ranging work in therapeutic recreation in general, led the National Committee to enlist her help as the administrative director of the SCS project site. She in turn secured the services of a former student, Randy Routon, as the site team leader. Routon, an instructor in the Department of Recreation at TWU, has led workshops and given lecture/demonstrations throughout the Southwest in the use of creative arts techniques in therapeutic recreation.

Routon and Sherrill worked closely with Carol Fritze to get the NCAH project at the Special Care School off the ground. And to make up at least part of the arts team there, they drew on the talents of some of their graduate students at Texas Woman's University.

The Roger Walton Development Center
The Walton Development Center is located on the northwest edge of Stockton, a middle-sized city that sits in central California's fertile San Joaquin Valley some 50 miles below Sacramento. It shares grounds with a high school named for the legendary College (now University) of the Pacific football coach Alonzo Stagg.

Walton Center is administered by the Stockton Unified School District on funds derived mainly from local taxes. It was established in 1961, as the first Development Center in the state, to serve children who "have delayed development or mental retardation and are not eligible for any other public school programs." For years it has also provided University of the Pacific special education students with a kind of built-in "lab school."

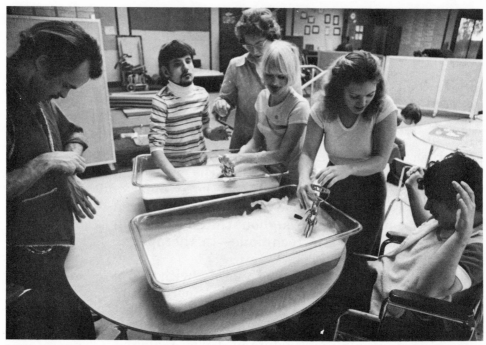

Walton teachers give children sensory and fine motor experiences (bubble-bath play, above, and papier-maché activity, below)

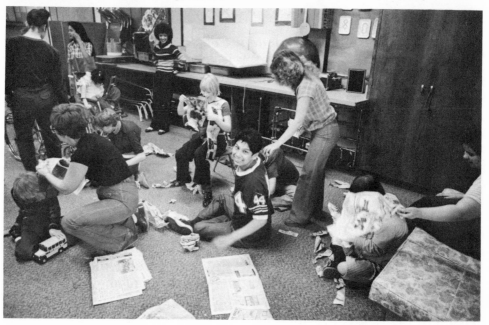

Its public school status is, of course, one way in which Walton differs from Great Oaks and SCS. Another more obvious way is that, instead of many small homeroom environments where quite limited numbers of children are taught by one or two teachers, the teaching at Walton takes place in three very large teaching spaces, each populated by perhaps three dozen children who are "team-taught" by a virtual corps of instructors.

Each of the classrooms is large enough to handle between thirty and forty youngsters. Movable furniture and other devices can be arranged to section off the space and make smaller isolated areas (even cubbyholes) when the staff needs to work "one on one" or with groups of two or three children. Several smaller rooms adjoin each classroom and can be used for these purposes too.

The teaching teams that work in these large spaces consist of perhaps ten or a dozen persons: several head teachers with aides to assist them plus the volunteers and practicum students who are on hand intermittently—and a few former students who have progressed to the TMR stage and can help with meals or toileting.

Although the equipment in these classrooms is similar in many ways to that in most Great Oaks and SCS classrooms, there is just a lot more of it scattered around: tables and chairs for meals or for game playing or academic work; waterbeds, plastic wedges, floppy beanbag chairs, and huge down-filled balls—all used for stimulating, handling, caring for, and exercising the nonambulatory kids; shelves of colorful and appropriate toys; carpeted spaces for dealing with the very young or the immobilized; room dividers; walls filled with posters, snapshots of the children, and progress charts—areas labeled "Language Center," "Perception Center," and "Gross Motor Center," with cards showing each child's progress toward specific objectives; and all manner of orthopedic equipment.

Aims and Goals of the Walton Program

The program at the Walton Center is planned to provide experiences that will enable severely handicapped children to develop abilities they possess to the fullest extent possible.

Children have the opportunities:

• *To develop and improve communicative skills, to express their needs and interests, to learn to listen, and to respond to others*

• *To learn to control their behavior according to acceptable standards and to practice habits of cleanliness, health, and eating so that they are not offensive when observed by others*

• *To improve sensory discrimination and coordination and to develop self-help skills such as feeding and dressing*

• *To learn to follow directions and to accept supervision*

• *To learn to get along with others, to take turns, and to participate in group activities*

• *To participate in satisfying and enjoyable experiences so essential to the development of good mental health*

Parents have opportunities:

• *To have some relief from the constant demands of caring for severely handicapped children, thus enabling them to be more efficient in their efforts when they are with their children*

• *To discuss their problems concerning their handicapped children with other parents, Development Center teachers, and persons working with the center as consultants*

• *To learn more about the various community resources which may be available to help them plan realistically for their severely handicapped children*

• *To work cooperatively with others interested in the welfare of the handicapped in effecting legislation and in developing further programs and services*

The Walton Center is designed so that all three teaching spaces are housed in an L-shaped building around a central court. Across the court, with connecting covered walk areas, is an administration building.

Another building south of the complex completes the center facilities, and what you come upon in this building is calculated to melt the hearts of even such celebrated children–haters as W.C. Fields. This structure houses Walton's Delayed Development Unit and its Home Training Unit, both of them programs geared to the needs of developmentally delayed children from birth to 3 years of age. These children were not included in the NCAH project because they were too young, but Roger and I managed to find our way there on more than one occasion to watch this utterly beguiling roomful of children crawling about on the floor and being ministered to by a special group of caring teachers.

For the three other classroom units, containing our project children, the length of the school day was similar to that at the other sites, beginning around 9:00 in the morning and ending at 3:00 or so in the afternoon. Parents were generally in evidence at Walton too (although perhaps not as much as at SCS). Some drive their children to school and come back to pick them up in the afternoons, but for the most part Walton students are transported in Stockton school system buses with the usual adaptations for handicapped riders.

The classroom units themselves are organized so that each contains groupings of children who represent, within certain rough age-spans, related kinds of handicapping conditions. Virtually all Walton students are in the severe or profound categories— but in Unit II, for instance, one finds almost all the nonambulatory kids between the ages of 3 and 12. In Unit III, most students are walking though they're not always fully coordinated, and they range in age from 12 through adolescence to 21. Unit I is for ambulatory kids from 3 to 12 who generally have longer attention spans but, at the same time, may exhibit more behavioral problems and need more control.

Serving as the administrative team at the California site were the director and a staff member at the Alan Short Center, a unique "cultural center for the handicapped" in Stockton. Established in 1976 in a roomy mansion on the grounds of the Stockton State Hospital, the Alan Short Center provides intensive training for mentally retarded and physically handicapped adults in both the visual and the performing arts. "Although 'therapy' plays an important part in the overall structure," Director Alan Falstrau points out, "our program in the arts has been designed to explore the talents and creativity of each individual."

Most of those who come for classes at the Alan Short Center function at the higher levels of retardation—the so-called mild or moderate categories. Groups of Alan Short Center students (the Short Swingers, a square-dancing ensemble, for example) have performed for and with their more severely handicapped friends at the Walton Center on a number of occasions.

Falstrau, whose center has been named an Arts for the Handicapped National Model Site by NCAH, was asked to take on the job of site administrative director. A graduate of the University of the Pacific, Falstrau had taught and worked professionally in theater. He engaged as site team leader, Yvonne Soto, a UCLA music major who went on to take advanced work at Cal State, Long Beach, and moved to Stockton to complete her music therapy internship at the Alan Short Center, where she teaches guitar. The project at Walton emerged from their joint planning and scheduling with the Center's Executive Director, Ann Trujillo.

3

SPECIAL CHILDREN, SPECIAL TEACHERS

WHEN YOU FIRST ENCOUNTER children as badly damaged in mind and body as most SPH kids are, you have the uneasy feeling that an unaccountable slippage has occurred along some plane of human existence—a time warp perhaps—and that you have, indeed, stepped into another world.

Partly it's the shock of seeing so many such children in one place all at once, riding down the bus lifts in their wheelchairs and crowding the patios and, later on, scattered through the classrooms. Partly, too, it's the incredible communication gap that exists between you—at first, at any rate. You expect to have problems communicating with an infant or a very young child. You don't expect them with a 10-year-old or a boy or girl in late adolescence. It's a shock to be confronted suddenly with so little comprehension in their faces, such complete neglect of the ordinary niceties, such intense and dedicated a response to invisible impulses—the children fill many of these rooms with human noises, but little human speech. And finally it's the pain you feel for them, because the damage inflicted on their minds and bodies has left them so helpless, so vulnerable.

Seeing these children in three separate schools, one after another, you wonder again with some rea-

The Small-Scale Changes

It's the small-scale changes that delight you. Like in Regina, who had always moved around by squirming along the floor. One day we see her on all fours and we realize she's been doing this crawling movement all along—but not in school for some reason. We tried to figure out how to keep her doing it, but nothing worked until we used her lunch plate. Regina is deaf—but we'd show her where we'd put that plate, on the table about 20 feet from her—and sure enough, that kid solved that problem. She crawled over to the table to get it. It's the only crawling she'll do though. We can't get her to crawl for anything else.

Little Mario—most of the time he just lies on one of the green beds with his head flopped down. He can't sit upright alone at all. But we've worked with him for a year now and if I sit behind him and prop his head up, he can now sit alone for one full second. To us, that's a great deal of progress.

We have some children, though, for whom we really can't set any goals—beyond what they're already doing. A child whose leg can bend just this far . . . if we can just maintain that action for her and not have her lose any ground so that the leg becomes stiffer—that can be a kind of goal in itself.

Kathy Saylor
Head Teacher in Unit II
Walton Development Center

son whether anything at all—much less the infusion of artistic elements into their world—can possibly enhance the quality of their lives or improve the ways they customarily function.

"Special" is a word you come to accept as definitive when it is applied to handicapped people—and especially to these SPH kids. As a group they are set apart from the rest of us for reasons they can not help, distinct among humans in a way that erases all other distinctions. I like the dictionary phrase "surpassing what is common or usual." Exceptional.

My colleague, Roger Vaughan, wrote *this* about these children after our initial visits: "The specialness begins with a remarkable absence of social inhibitions. . . . . The private and public posture of these children is the same. They are naked, special for their innocence, special for what they have *not* been able to learn or acquire."

At the same time, you come gradually to realize that there are crucial distinctions within that specialness. Although they function within a very narrow range, developmentally speaking, these children are as diverse in behavior, character, and personality as the rest of us. There is shyness among them, and openness, even directness; there is intensity in one, inertia in another; there is evident pain in the gaze of some, a clear bump of humor in the glance of others. Within their special world, there is, then, an extraordinary spectrum of individuality—as in *our* world. The point is, once again, that we don't expect to find it in their—and one of the many delights of the familiarization process is having them confound that naïve expectation.

Another early pleasure is when you find yourself acquiring the terminology. Suddenly you realize that you've moved past your early bewilderment with the basic professional jargon and are even using it (a bit self-consciously) yourself more and more. A few examples:

• Words like "attend," where the meaning is closer to the French *attendez*, meaning "to pay attention." ("Just getting Carrie to attend," a teacher will say, "is a good 20 minutes' work!")

• Phrases like "seriously involved," meaning not only "entangled" but something akin to "disabled in the extreme" and often used to describe a *multiple* handicap (as in Ann Trujillo's comment about Walton's Unit II children: "When kids are this seriously involved, they're not just retarded, they have another handicap as well, maybe several. They may be retarded *plus* have cerebral palsy *plus* suffer from seizures—or maybe they don't see and hear very well and have a great deal of sensory deprivation").

• Phrases like "inappropriate behavior" or "unacceptable behavior" which have particular meaning when, for instance, a tall boy of 16 with mouth agape comes up to you and says "hello" loudly with his face 3 or 4 inches from yours.

• A term like "functioning level," which isn't a bad way at all to talk about the actions and behaviors that characterize specific stages of human development.

Happily there is a time early on in one's indoctrination when it becomes clear that the words "severely" and "profoundly" are not merely descriptive adjectives chosen at random but specific categories of handicap and retardation. They, in effect, define two discrete functioning levels at the low end of the scale. So—when a teacher says, "He's a very low functioning child," you can feel fairly certain she's speaking of a *profoundly* handicapped child. And it is implied, therefore, that "higher functioning" refers to the *severe* level of retardation.

But that's not quite accurate either. Because when teachers make distinctions between children in the *same* category, they'll be apt to say that "Claire is higher functioning than Molly." It seems to depend on which of the two levels you're on when you start making such comparisons.

At one point in my early encounters with these children, I had a flash of insight that I felt could be applied to this matter of functioning levels in order to clarify the subtleties.

From what we'd been told, I had the impression that none of these children was functioning much above a 3-year-old level. To bring that point to life, I tried to remember what my own children were like during the years when they were between 18 months and 3 years old. I tried to recall as clearly as I could what my children knew at that age; how they learned (or were trained); how they behaved alone, or in groups; when, for instance, they learned to manipulate a crayon (fine motor ability) and to ride a trike (gross motor); how they ate and drank and communicated with us; and what pleased them and what annoyed them.

It seemed to me that this mechanism might help me place these children in better perspective. Certainly, I thought, it could help me translate into personal terms the activities and behaviors of a classroom of children whose chronological ages ranged through adolescence, for example. Of course, it wasn't easy even then to disassociate the way they *looked* from the kinds of developmental behavior they exhibited. But the mechanism helped for a time . . . until a teacher at Great Oaks named Marlene Becker* gave me a piece of information that modified even this device.

Marlene was telling me about Elmer, an earnest and hypertense youth of 20 and a member of her class of older students requiring modified behavior-management techniques. Elmer is listed as profoundly retarded. But his behavior didn't fit my static picture of a 3-year-old. Then I learned that Elmer, in fact, functioned at *different* age levels depending on which developmental characteristic you were talking about.

Marlene pointed out that Elmer was functioning at the 4-year-old level in "self-care skills" according to the behavior scale employed at Great Oaks; he had learned to button, zip, and buckle his own clothes. He was, however, on the 2½-year-old level in language development ("he knows many signs but

*Marlene Becker received the NCAH Outstanding Educator Award on June 26, 1979, in ceremonies at the John F. Kennedy Center in Washington.

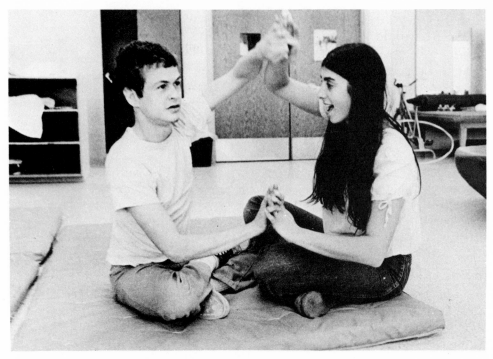

Elmer with Marlene Becker. (Photo by Molly A. Roberts)

uses only a few"). And he was functioning on the
3-year-old level in social skills ("he'll play by himself, but he often slips into stereotyped behaviors
such as rocking his body and waving his hands"). In
fine-motor-skill development, he functioned at a
4-year-old level ("but poor attending, and hand
tremors make many fine motor tasks difficult for
him"), and he functioned at the 4½-year-old level in
gross motor skills ("his strongest area of functioning"). And finally, Elmer functioned on the 3-year-
old level in cognitive skills ("he can identify objects
by name using sign language . . . learning his sex is
a goal for Elmer this year—he will be able to sign
that he is a boy before too long").

So here before me was a 20-year-old boy (almost a
man) whose behaviors in six different developmental areas varied from that of a child of 2½ to

one of 4½. Once again, the lesson seemed to be that you can't categorize rigidly about human lives and behaviors in these children. There are no immutable certainties, no labels that can be applied in hard and fast terms. They are individuals and they can't be typed inflexibly; they vary as unpredictably as the nonretarded or the nonhandicapped across the continuum of qualities and conditions that make us all human.

Then, also at Great Oaks, there was Eugenia. In Eugenia, who weighs 27 pounds and is confined to a wheelchair, you are suddenly caught up by the enigma of a 13-year-old girl who in most respects functions at a *3-month-old* level of development. Because of her profound physical involvement, however, her fine and gross motor abilities could not be assigned a developmental age. "She can turn her head from side to side very slightly," her teacher Joanne Campell told me. "Her hands are usually closed, and they can be made to relax and open only if you manipulate them. She doesn't have any reflex grasping, leg, trunk, or arm movements."

In the area of self-help, Eugenia is about at the 3-month level. "She's able to suck pureed food from a spoon and drink from a cup that's held for her," Joanne said. "She doesn't gag or choke when she swallows, but often she'll make kind of a snoring noise while breathing."

In the social, language, and cognitive areas, Eugenia scores at the 3-month level as well. But Joanne pointed out that she has a high degree of visual awareness, she is very responsive to people, and she watches most of what goes on around her.

This piece of information gives one pause. As does this: "Eugenia will track a person from one end of the room to another," Joanne continued. "She will attend to and track objects—but she prefers to track people. She'll smile, look directly at a speaker's face, and she often makes an 'ah' sound when she's happy. She generally responds pleasantly to familiar persons and social approaches."

These things aren't always apparent until you get to know children like Eugenia better—and even then you may need to watch carefully for the signs. But when you do spot them, when one of these children who seems so dull, listless, and immobile does look directly at you and smiles, you know a very special kind of joy. And even in those children who may never respond overtly—never show any interest or express themselves in any way—you learn that this doesn't necessarily mean there's no comprehension or understanding taking place at some level.

In this special human arena, the traditional milestones of progress are scaled down to quarter inches or less.

I am standing in the Multiage Training Class at the Special Care School looking down at Maria. It is a December day, the week of our first visit there. Maria and the other five children in this class are virtually immobilized by their handicaps. Maria is very frail; her tiny hands are clenched awkwardly at her sides, her lips drawn (in pain, I wonder?), and she is lying back almost motionless on a green plastic wedge at my feet. She appears to be perhaps 5 or 6 years old, but I have already learned not to judge these children's ages by their bodies and faces.

As Roger wrote later: "Their faces are rare, open, ageless, misplaced. . . . To paraphrase the poet Theodore Roethke, something is amiss when a child of three can wear an ancient face."

I am unable to make eye contact with Maria. In fact, I am not even certain she is aware of me at all. And I wonder what the *quality* of this child's life must be like, whether her mind holds any thoughts at all or her psyche any feelings? Can there be valid human purpose to life imprisoned in such a body as hers?

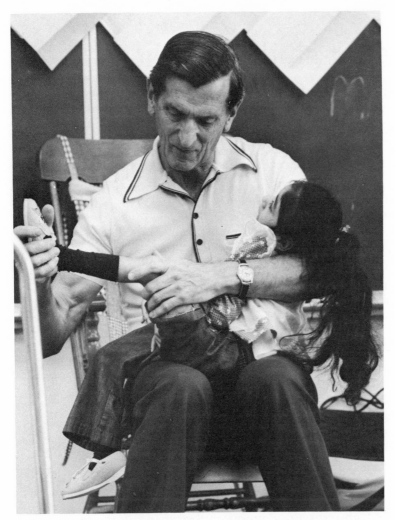

Harold Rettig, SCS custodian/artist, working with Maria.

Suddenly I am aware that someone has come up beside me—a man with greying hair and a good, keen face whom I've seen around the school, more often than not working with the children. We squat down and he picks up Maria's clenched hands and begins gently to massage them. He talks softly to her for awhile and finally her eyes seek his face. He turns to me and says, "You know, when Maria first

"The Possibility Is There . . ."

*In the years I've been here, we've had so many breakthroughs—
and those are the things you keep remembering, the things you
keep hoping for every day. Like Cheryl. I've worked with her for
four or five years now. Even the doctors said Cheryl'd never be
anything . . . just a vegetable, really. She was growing into a
ball almost, with her knees up against her chest.*

*Well, we've all worked with her, year after year. I've walked her
and exercised her everyday. I had her yesterday to the point
where she placed her weight on her feet and was almost ready to
push herself up and take off—with some help of course. But
somebody has to keep at it; first thing we put her in a walker,
she'll start to bend. So you have to keep working. But I hope that
eventually Cheryl is going to walk. We don't know, but the possibility is there.*

Harold Rettig
Inside Custodian
Special Care School

came here a year or so ago, she was practically a
vegetable, seemed like. But *now* . . . she's doing just
fine . . . developing a real personality of her own."

I learned later that day that he was Harold Rettig,
a retired steelworker who'd come south from
Pittsburgh a few years earlier and taken on the job of
"indoor custodian" at SCS because he loved to be
around these children and work with them when he
had time. He turned out to be an artist, as well, a
portrait artist—and a carpenter; he'd built most of
the homemade orthopedic devices I'd seen around
the school. Someone told me he also kept personal
journals on many of the children.

His comment about Maria nudged me past one of
the hang-ups that persist for awhile when you're
first in the presence of such children. You ask your-

self, "What's the use? Why bother to train them at all?" Obviously, Harold Rettig knew why—from experience: he could see something happening in Maria, over time; changes that, however incremental and however long in coming, were evidence of the humanity she'd been unable to reveal or express until now. That was all the reason one needed to become committed to this cause, to keep working at it regardless.

Indeed, as Louise Appell put it, "you don't end up teaching damaged children unless you believe you can effect change—and you must learn to be satisfied with almost imperceptible bits of evidence to tell you change has taken place." Clearly, the teachers in these schools and those on the support staffs, like Harold Rettig, would also affirm her fundamental contention that "no level of human activity is so deficient as to preclude learning."

There appears to be little more precision in this field than in many other professions today. The intelligence quotient, for instance, has long been one of the factors that professionals use to define these populations. The *severely* handicapped person has often been "defined" as one who has an IQ of between 20 and 35, and the *profoundly* handicapped an IQ of less than 20. But these figures are apt to be no more valid as the sole measure for determining placement of a child in special classes than the higher numbers would be in the regular world of schooling.

The same could be said about discrete behaviors and characteristics. The severely handicapped are often said to be characterized by self-stimulation, self-mutilation, aggression toward others, severe sensory or physical defects, poor communication skills, and so on. Those in the profound category, meanwhile, are said to have only a few reflexes, extreme feeding problems, inability to sit erect, and numerous associated disorders.

While all of this may indeed be true, it isn't enough to satisfy some authorities.* They are challenging such definitions today as being much too simplistic and, particularly, as "lacking in relevance for educational programming." There are echoes here, in fact, of that complaint we often hear voiced in regular schools—a failure to deal with *the whole child*. And it's leading these authorities to question the use of finite numbers and static definitions in all areas of special education. They make it clear that "defining, labeling, and categorizing have little point unless they lead specifically to appropriate educational placement and programming." It would seem to be clear as well that this aspect of special education is still in its early formative stages—and that a great deal more research and development work remains to be done.

To bring about progress of any kind in an SPH child's learning life, his teachers will encourage, cajole, drill, tease, and play with him day after day—just as parents and teachers do with normal kids they're guiding through the first 3 years of life. But the learning here takes place over a greatly stretched-out time span—and it is charted in terms of short-term and long-term goals prescribed for each child in the IEP, or individual educational plan.

The specific objectives vary from child to child, obviously, but at lower functioning levels they might include toilet training and learning to eat with a spoon and drink from a cup; word imitation (bye-bye, Mommy and Daddy, and hi); identifying body parts; responding to a "come here" command; discriminat-

---

*McDowell and Sontag, "The Severely and Profoundly Handicapped as Catalysts for Change," in *Educational Programming for the Severely and Profoundly Handicapped*, published by the Division of Mental Retardation, The Council for Exceptional Children, pp. 3-5, 1977.

SPH: Some Definitions

The NCAH Project relied on a broad, educationally oriented definition (established by the BEH) to help each site designate which children should be included in the project.

It identified as severely and profoundly handicapped those children who are "seriously emotionally disturbed, with extreme mental retardation, and those having two or more serious handicapping conditions—the mentally retarded blind, for instance, and the cerebral-palsied deaf."

More specifically, such children would be characterized by any or all of the following: "severe language and/or perceptual-cognitive deprivations . . . failure to respond to pronounced social stimuli . . . self-mutilation . . . self-stimulation . . . intense and prolonged temper tantrums . . . absence of rudimentary forms of verbal control . . . severely fragile psychological conditions."

ing between two objects (cup and spoon perhaps); and standing alone without falling.

At the higher functioning levels, with youngsters in the severe category (some of whom may even be approaching the trainable stage), the objectives become less infantile, more cognitive in nature: telling time by the hour, identifying coins, talking out loud, learning to use the phone (dialing numbers, answering questions like "Who's this?" and "Where are you?"), and other social (and survival) skills.

The nonverbal or language-delayed children in both of these low-functioning categories are generally taught to "sign" in order to make their wants known, often combining the sign language with any verbalizations that occur.

The children, for their part, become quite adept at pulling all the traditional stratagems of the nonhandicapped 2-, 3-, or 4-year-old to gain atten-

On Teachers of the Retarded

What makes a good teacher in this field? Well, traditionally, people used to say that it takes patience. And I guess it does—but to me the most important thing of all is a sense of humor. You have to enjoy living and try not to take life so seriously.

You've got to be able to laugh—at yourself, at those kids, and at the whole ridiculous situation you and they are in. That's what keeps us going. If you're too involved with the kids, or their families, if you're too intense and too dedicated, it catches up with you in the end. So a sense of humor ... well, it just goes with the territory.

Then—you have to be able to think on your feet ... be aware of what's going on around you all the time ... and quick to respond. But this needs to be combined with that element of patience they used to stress, because development and growth and progress comes so incrementally in these children.

I look for people who are creative too. Dependable. Resourceful. People who see what needs to be done and go ahead and do it.

If candidates for a job here tell me in an interview that they've never had a student they didn't like, I don't believe it. They really aren't

tion, win approval, or get their own way. They wheedle, tease, stall, pretend they didn't hear, feign attacks and illnesses, and—as the teachers say— "just plain manipulate us to death if they possibly can."

The *causes* of the afflictions suffered by the SPH child are almost without exception beyond the child's control: brain damage at birth, rubella, Apert's Disease (resulting in webbed fingers and toes), Down's syndrome, cerebral palsy, genetic deficiencies, and many which are simply labeled as "etiology unknown." At first, one is convinced that it being honest when they say that. Each of these teachers here has favorites. If there's ever anybody who has a deep antipathy toward a kid, we'll try to change the situation, of course—but I have real difficulty with the premise that simply because a child is retarded, you should ipso facto *like* him. Some are cute and adorable and others are just as ornery as can be. It's just not possible for you to feel the same about each child. Sure, you have compassion and you care about them . . . but that's separate from "liking."

Carol Fritze
Director
Special Care School

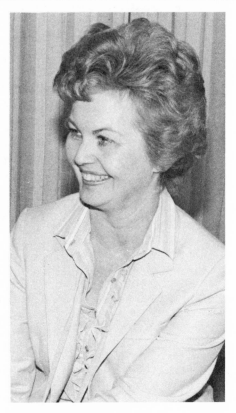

Carol Fritze. (Photo by Rae Allen)

is equally beyond their control to do anything at all about their situation. But gradually you realize that most of them *can* do something about it, when they're helped by their parents (if they live with their families) *and* by their teachers.

Perhaps especially it is the teachers who can make the difference. They work with the children for a concentrated 6-hour period each weekday, and they often take time after that to counsel with parents, encouraging them to work in similar ways at home when they have the chance. It is difficult, painstaking work—with every one of the senses attuned to what the children in their charge are doing every minute of the time. And, for those teachers who must deal with children who cannot move without help (including some with large, rapidly maturing bodies), it is, quite literally, backbreaking work.

As a group, the teachers and aides who work with SPH kids tend to be young women. They invariably seem to possess vibrancy and energy. For the most part, they are a highly articulate, generally alert, and cheerful group of people—quick to laugh, quick to act when the need arises, generally "up front" with their feelings.

Men serve as classroom aides at the Walton Center, but there were only two men among the head teachers at the three schools; slightly less vibrant perhaps and more diffident than their female colleagues, but with much the same energy and alertness, they were both in charge of highly structured "behavior mod" classrooms.

Interestingly enough, *these* classrooms—where considerable strength and force is often required—were not the exclusive province of men. Women were assigned to them also, some as aides assisting the men but others as head teachers with no men in their rooms. It was startling sometimes to see these young women move quickly into action and apply the force required to bring an unruly or insensate youngster under control.

Aside from their special education training and their knowledge of child growth and development, what seemed to characterize these teachers (men and women alike) most strongly was their refreshing combination of caring and tough-mindedness. It seemed to be grounded in their sense of humor, or at least in their sense of the ridiculous. It was also grounded in the successful resolution most of them made of two powerful but conflicting human impulses: their deep compassionate feelings for these children (even for the kids who weren't among their favorites) and their equally strong commitment to professional objectivity.

Sure—we play favorites. You can't help it. But there's somebody for everybody. Each kid seems to have somebody who treats him special . . . who cares more for him than for any of the others. And sometimes the rest of us can't figure out why. So—you have to work real hard with everybody, but you don't have to love everybody.

Lynn Johnson
Education Supervisor
Great Oaks Center

This loving toughness, this tempering of sentiment with professionalism comes out most readily in their alertness to situations in which a child may be "manipulating" them—and their refusal to fall for any of the tricks that may be used on them. Or at least *attempting* to keep the practice under control, not to be fooled by it too often or lulled too readily into indulging their favorites.

"You really don't help these kids by letting them get away with murder," is the way a Walton teacher put it. "We've always got to keep in mind that one of these days, if he isn't totally immobilized, maybe—just *maybe*—that kid's going to advance far enough to move into the trainable category. And that means he's got to be as independent as possible. We're doing him no kindness to let him get around us all the time, because that just means he'll delay learning how to get along without us until maybe it's too late."

Their loving toughness comes out also in their somewhat sardonic humor and their fond mockery of their kids. Angela Blatchley, a teacher at Great Oaks, tried for some time to get a small, partly sighted boy named Joe to react to a perky hand puppet as we sat watching. But he took no notice, made no response. Then, after we'd moved into the hall, out of sight, I heard Angie laugh and say with jovial reproval, "Oh, I see—*now* you're gonna do it, aren't you? Just like a little *regular* child!" And she didn't call us back in to tell us about this either.

They're all tremendously proud of their kids, too. Marlene, at Great Oaks, indicated just how much when she owned up to some empathetic stage fright for Elmer and the rest of her class; for some weeks they'd been rehearsing their "act" for the Very Special Arts Festival that would climax the arts project in June. "I know it's the process, not the product that's important," Marlene told me, "but I really, really hope they do well tomorrow. It's not for me—*I* know they can do these things, but a lot of other people may not—and I just want them to show people how really good they are!"

These SPH teachers are also prone to something that occurs at some point in almost every good teacher's career—the syndrome they refer to as "burnout." It is perhaps more prevalent among teachers of handicapped youngsters, however, for all the obvious reasons. "You get to a point," a teacher at Great Oaks said, "where you don't feel you have any more to offer the kids—you've drained yourself, worn yourself out, emotionally and physically. Maybe mentally, too. You need to get away for a time and refresh yourself when this comes over you. For a lot of us, it hits sometime around the fifth or sixth year of teaching. Some people decide to take a sabbatical or something when burnout time comes. but a lot of times they end up leaving the field entirely."

Special children—special teachers. You come to know them fairly well, you think, after being around them for 3 or 4 days the first time you visit one of the schools. You're on a first-name basis very quickly with the teachers, and you identify the children that way too. . . . Chucky and Lori and Jamie and Chris. By the time you leave, you've pretty well got the names and the faces tied together in your mind.

But you move on to the next project site, and then to a third, playing the same kind of identification

An Institutionalized Child

Holly likes to do challenging things, but she's also very snobbish. You have to like her usually before she likes you. She watches people's reactions to her—she has partial sight and partial hearing—and people will say, "Oh, she's so stubborn, and so snobbish, and so this and that." Now, actually, she is all of those things to a degree, but that's what makes her such an interesting personality.

Here she is, a little 10-year-old institutionalized child who's severely retarded, who knows that someone is going to take care of her and respond to all her needs—and she really does know that. Take her Dressing Program for example—she acts like you're really stepping on her toes to expect her to dress herself because she knows she's dressed every morning by the staff back in her unit. So she's really asking why would we be doing something as silly as trying to have her dress herself in the classroom. That's how smart she is.

I tend to push her a bit as a result, and she lets people she likes a lot push her some. A little risk-taking thing I do with her now is to stand her in a corner where she can brace herself, put a big beanbag next to her and encourage her to fall over it, to let herself go. And she usually does, with no fear and much delight. What this shows is that she doesn't mind working or taking risks if she feels it's interesting enough to be worth her while. If it's real dull, like dressing herself, she won't do it.

Angie Blatchley
Teacher
Great Oaks Center

games—and when you return again to the first school a month or 6 weeks later, you find you have to start all over again learning which names go with all those familiar faces.

Partly, we came to feel, it's because there is a curious similarity among the inhabitants of these schools—teachers and children alike. Among the teachers it's more a matter of attitude and energy level than appearance, perhaps, but there does seem to be a certain type of active and caring young person who is drawn to this kind of teaching. Among the children, though, it's a matter of appearance almost entirely: there are counterparts in each place to the Elmers, the Marias, the Cheryls, and the Eugenias. Their respective handicapping conditions seem to produce remarkable likenesses in the way these children appear—and this is certainly one of the more obvious ways in which their specialness manifests itself.

Most of the teachers, it happens, had very little background in the arts. The colleges they attended to obtain their B.A.'s in special education haven't generally placed much value on the arts for prospective teachers of handicapped youngsters. So the educational potential of the arts is largely overlooked, either as experiences through which to explore one's own creativity or as resources to be used as a teaching tool. As a result, the handicapped child has little chance to be exposed to or become involved in the world of the arts. Except for what any good early childhood teacher does to liven up her classroom environment, and the occasional appearance of an art or music therapist, the arts are often as neglected in these special schools as they are in educational programs in general.

During the life of this NCAH Project, however, that situation was drastically altered for the special teachers and special children in the three pilot schools, as some equally special people called artists entered into and variously affected their world.

AN INFUSION OF ARTISTS

Walton Center, November 1978

THE LARGE TEACHING space known as Unit II at the Walton Development Center has been rearranged for a meeting. Nearly fifty folding chairs have been placed in a circle on one side of the room. Some are already occupied and the conversational pitch is rising. The 6-foot 6-inch frame of puppeteer George Latshaw towers amiably over several Walton teachers who stand chatting with him near the door.

It is a warm day in late November 1978, and the room is slowly filling up with the expected mix of people who will shortly be working in and around the SPH arts project in Stockton: teachers, administrators, teacher aides, volunteers, some parents, and members of the local Arts Team who will be working in Walton classrooms over the months ahead. They are all gathering for the second of three afternoon workshops Latshaw is conducting to launch the new NCAH venture.

Latshaw is indeed an extremely tall man with an imposing presence and an angular, rough-hewn face. Sensitive and unassuming, he looks at the world thoughtfully (and often humorously) through dark-rimmed spectacles. He has an easy rambling manner of speaking and his entire demeanor is warm and enormously reassuring. His reputation as a puppeteer and a performing artist is, of course, worldwide; a former president of Puppeteers of America, he has worked in both motion pictures and television and has, many times over the years,

49

brought the worlds of puppetry and theater closer together. Most often it has been through the medium of children's theater, an environment where his puppets have been most at home.

As the project's so-called principal artist, Latshaw is responsible for setting much of the operational tone for this endeavor, for giving it some broad directional cues, and for providing it with a kind of philosophic underpinning. The NCAH staff refer to him as "a catalyst" and that may indeed capture much of the essence of his role; he hopes in any event, to "precipitate" the process by means of the workshop sequence he's designed as an orientation vehicle. It is a 3-day sequence he will refine here and then repeat (with possible modifications) next week at the Special Care School in Dallas, and again at the Great Oaks Center in Maryland the following week.

Yesterday's session was the opener and both Louise Appell and Ralph Nappi from the National Committee were on hand to express their hopes for the project and place it in perspective within the NCAH framework. Louise Appell told the group:

There's no need to remind you that an undertaking like this doesn't happen by magic. This is something that's never been tried before, anywhere, on this scale, so we're pioneering here and it's going to take a lot of very dedicated work on the part of everyone involved to give it a fair chance. Many of the good things will happen simultaneously—the old "A-ha" light will flash in the same way in each place, I guarantee it. But it's a valuable undertaking no matter what the outcomes are. In my guts, though, I know it's going to work.

Latshaw had geared that first day's workshop toward encouraging the project people—and teachers in particular—to let down their hair a little and begin exploring their own creative and imaginative processes. Working in pairs or in small groups, they were led through exercises that helped them to communicate using pantomime, to improvise dra-

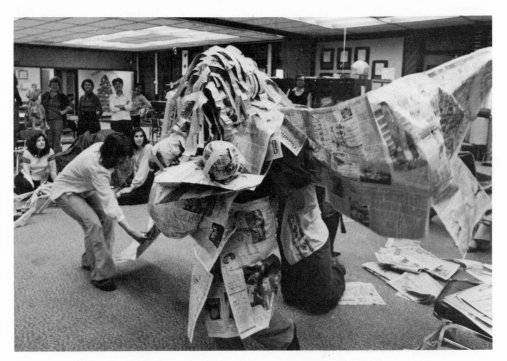

Teachers at a Walton workshop session create a papier-maché dragon.

matic plots in a very short time, and to create fanciful animals and complex machines using only stacks of old newspapers and some paper tape. He told them:

All of these exercises are aimed at making you realize the creative process isn't limited to an elite group of people somewhere called artists. *Everyone* has that capacity within them to create—it's unique and individual. And it's only by *doing* it here like this and finding it's joyous and exciting that, out of that joy, you can grow to the point where you're not afraid to take another risk—and then another. We're trying to pull out of you those things that are part of your life experience and make you what you are—the qualities that *you* have and no one else in this room has. Let's get those creative juices flowing so we can start putting the blocks together and gradually, step by step, build this process model the National Committee has asked us to bring into being.

Imaging With Children

Puppets have so much to offer a child in terms of what I call "imaging." They give you a positive way for developing in children a deep sense of nurture or caring toward the puppet—it's like a pet or a living thing that's smaller than they are, but whose response can be controlled. A puppet can be anything, really, that's animated by human control.

The dancing or moving finger puppets have particular appeal to deaf children because they recognize the action doesn't require speech—and *they* use their fingers to communicate, too, when they're signing.

Tempo is important in puppetry with these children. We can slow the movement down and get our character to be deliberate and graceful, or we can speed him up and get a kind of cartoonlike blur going "w-h-i-i-i-i-s-s-h-h."

The marvelous thing is that the magic of illusion exists, whether you *see* the person who's animating the puppet or not. It isn't because the animator is *hidden*, it's in his believing that can make an illusion with the puppet. . . . By putting the focus on what the puppet is saying and doing, he establishes the puppet's own relationship with the audience.

With puppets we're cut loose from making those invidious comparisons with the real world. We are whatever we *want* to be . . . or can become! It's this new viewpoint—working away from reality—that gives the puppet *its real* life . . . it's independent, living in its own world, but it's still able to communicate with us.

To me, puppets have a strong therapeutic value because of this. When I was young, I wanted to be about 5-foot-6 and quick and lithe like the musical comedy performer Robert Morse. People would see me, though, and say, "Come on—knock it off—it's too funny." But that didn't stop me from wanting to do or be that different kind of person—so I identify with puppets in therapeutic terms because, for me, they've performed that function. I can use this pair of white gloves and make them into a puppet, and this is my

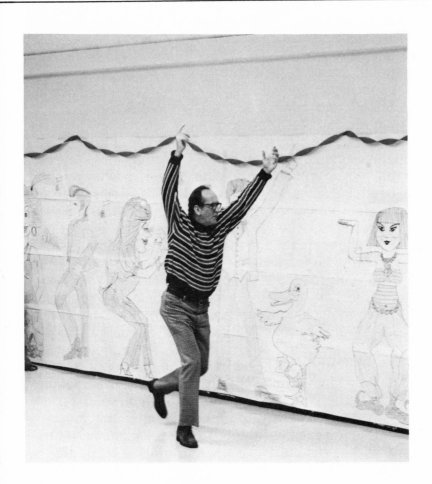

way of being Robert Morse,
or of being a little kitten or a
puppy and trying to get you
to go "A-w-w-w-w" the way
we do in response to things
that are small. I can be those
things and be this big tall
person named George too.

George Latshaw

During today's session Latshaw will focus mainly
on the ways his own creativity has expressed itself.
He plans to talk about his philosophy of puppetry
and why he has found that his particular art form
lends itself so compellingly to work with handicapped youngsters. He has brought along from his
home (and operating base) in Ohio a trunkful of
simple but fascinating puppet characters he's created quite literally out of whole cloth: fabrics,
gloves, paper cups and plates, buttons, drawer pulls,
plaster, styrofoam, and even a section of dryer hose
(that becomes an inchworm). He's given them all
distinctive voices and actions, of course, and he will
show us how the various members of his puppet family behave and what they're capable of doing.

Then, tomorrow, his demonstrations will take a
different turn, as puppets and children meet one
another for the first time. While the artists and
teachers look on, Latshaw will bring into each of the
classrooms in turn several of his simplest hand puppets: a prancing white-glove finger puppet, a flop-
eared hound-dog hand puppet, and a perky, matter-
of-fact lad named Wilbur whose head is a small
styrofoam ball stuck on the end of a dowel.

Working his way patiently around the room, he
will bring each child face to face with one or another
of these puppets and see what kinds of responses occur. Although he worked briefly with SPH kids last
spring at Great Oaks, this is relatively new territory
to Latshaw; he says he's not at all sure what—if
anything—will happen. But his performance career
has made him a risk taker and an experimenter,
qualities he and the other artists will draw on continually as the project proceeds.

"This relationship of performer to audience," he
says now, "is always a chancy thing, an unknown,
whether it's 200 children in a theater or on a one-
to-one basis with a kid in a classroom. With youngsters like these, especially, we just have to go with it
and see what the limits are. Their response will
suggest what I feel I ought to do next. And that im-

pulsive, spontaneous way of working is the fun *I* get out of it. I hope you'll find that to be true for you as well."

By the time these orientation workshops have run their course, it is clear that Latshaw has no artistic blueprint whatsoever up his sleeve when it comes to working with these children. He will himself be looking for answers, for productive ways of working, and he'll be going through a trial-and-error process with the kids in his own art form—so he will expect no more than this of anyone else. What he has hoped to do in the workshops is to provide both teachers and artists with a kind of launching pad, a creative springboard they could use to activate their own ideas and approaches during his absences. And he's also tried to create a climate in which constructive working relationships can develop between artists and teachers.

The artists, for their part, make a real attempt to reassure the teachers in each of the sites that they don't have any answers either; they'll be experimenting, too, they say, finding out what seems to work and what doesn't—and trying their best to help teachers work toward some of the objectives they've set for their children, not running counter to them or adding new goals of their own.

Despite such reassurances, an undercurrent of apprehension (and some skepticism as well) is evident among some members of each school's faculty. In a sense, the situation fits the classic mold; it has, for over a decade now, been encountered frequently in regular public schools when attempts have been made to "utilize arts resources" that exist beyond the schoolhouse doors. Usually, it is not the classroom teachers who request such help; more often it is thrust upon them by well-meaning "outsiders" or their own administrators who are simply taking advantage of available government or foundation funding opportunities.

But, however it is brought about, the appearance of professional artists on the educational scene is seldom regarded by teachers as an unalloyed blessing, a propitious answer to all their teaching and learning problems. It goes deeper, even, than the probability that the "chemistry" somehow won't be right between the two—a supposedly uninhibited, unconventional force meeting a presumably uptight traditional object. It is simply the fact that one's defenses *naturally* go up when someone who may be qualified in another field but not in yours comes in out of nowhere and begins demonstrating to you how to do your job. Presumably (as you get the message) you have failed to incorporate something of extreme value in your daily teaching routine—and these more highly gifted outsiders can provide you with the missing ingredient. Whether or not this ultimately turns out to be the case, there is certainly a natural human response involved here.

It isn't helped, either, by the fact that more than a few of the artists who tread on educational turf do so (initially at least) in a manner that seems almost calculated to bring about such a response. There is frequently a kind of missionary zeal about their actions and behaviors reminiscent of those who have found The Way and are determined to save you whether you want to be saved or not. Moreover, because they generally possess the sort of dash and charisma that students admire, and because their ways of working are indeed apt to be more open and spontaneous than that of many teachers, they are often a hard act to follow when their temporary involvement with the school comes finally to an end. And end it ultimately will—leaving the teachers once again with the full-time responsibility for their children's education.

Unless, during the intervention period, a genuine effort is made by both sides of this human equation to act with some sensitivity and keep the lines of communication open, the productive partnerships inherent in these situations have a hard time emerging. When they do happen, of course, the children seldom remain untouched or go unrewarded.

Teachers of SPH kids may, however, be entitled to an even greater skepticism about the teaching and learning potential of the arts than their colleagues in regular schools. On the surface of it, the reasons are obvious: their children are the hardest of all to reach, the most difficult to elicit responses from, and (seemingly) the least likely to be much enriched by the elusive attributes of the arts per se; besides, there is so much to be accomplished that is seemingly more crucial to these children's very survival that it's hard to imagine finding time for such non-utilitarian pursuits. Carol Fritze put it this way:

When you have to spend your time on such basics as toilet training and feeding, let alone helping a 9-year-old kid learn to walk—when you're trying to teach some cognitive things, setting up goals and assessing progress on such microscopic levels, *plus* meeting with parents regularly, *plus* going to all the after-hours meetings—well, maybe it's understandable that these teachers are fearful that all these essentials are going to be compromised somehow, maybe placed on the back burner for 5 or 6 months, because suddenly we're going to do the arts.

There is certainly some of this feeling abroad; you sense it from site to site during the orientation sessions with George Latshaw. On the other hand, there also appears to be plenty of genuine teacher interest in the program, too—a feeling that it may give them something new and useful, a boost to their morale perhaps, something to counteract burnout and provide a sense of renewal. But it's a posture somewhere in the middle, a kind of interested but watchful wait-and-see attitude, that seems to predominate among the teachers as this first round of Latshaw workshops ends and the project activities begin in earnest.

Great Oaks, February 1979

It is February now and we have returned to Great Oaks to begin our second series of site visits. The four artists have been working here for nearly two months now and both Lynn Johnson, the education supervisor, and Jan Goodrich, the site team leader, tell us that already some worthwhile things have been happening. They show us copies of the weekly logs the teachers and the artists have been filling out that describe some of the activities, and they comment on their value. And they suggest we simply roam the building these next few days and see for ourselves what's underway.

The artists each spend a total of two half-days in the classrooms every week, with Friday mornings reserved for feedback discussion sessions with Jan. A schedule has been arranged for their classroom visits that is aimed at bringing them in contact with each of Great Oaks' 100 or so "project children" at least once each week. It is a schedule, obviously, that keeps the artists traveling in high gear during the 3 hours they're at the school—and it's especially pressurized for those team members who may occasionally want to remove children from the classroom to work with them individually or in smaller groups. (Because it is *truly* a breakneck pace and only gives them brief in-and-out times with the children each week, the schedules will very shortly be altered so that each child will indeed have time— more leisurely time—every week with one or more of the artists, but not necessarily with *all* four of them.)

So, together or separately but ready for almost anything, Roger Vaughan and I immerse ourselves for several days in this arts-impacted educational environment.

I turn a corner on the main floor of the school and come upon a person in striking kingly attire—a purple flowing robe, a golden vest, glittery moneybag, jeweled crown, and feathery scepter—moving majes-

*Some exciting responses have occurred with
many of the children that are, I think, related
basically to their beginning to recognize me.
Many of them enjoy—and, I believe,
understand—the "joke" when someone acts
"silly" in a costume. In this sense, I believe
they are able to grasp the abstract ideas behind
"theater." They enjoy characters who behave
"unusually" and I think, because of this role
playing we do, they're somehow able to distin-
guish the "drama period" from the other arts
activities.*

Janine Stone (Drama)
Great Oaks Arts Team

---

tically down the hall and blowing a very raucous
horn.

Several youngsters appear at the door of a classroom and watch excitedly as the King pauses before
them and says grandly, "The King summons you,
Michael! You must kneel and be knighted!" Michael
C., an aloof, often sad-looking boy in what looks to be
late adolescence, does indeed perk up and kneel in
the doorway before the King. The King taps him
gently on the shoulder with the scepter, dubs him
"Sir Michael," and they disappear into the classroom
together.

The King turns out to be a lively and uninhibited
young actress named Janine Stone who is the drama
person on the team. She has degrees in theater from
several universities, but she is playing roles at
Great Oaks she could hardly have envisioned back
in drama school. Later, she explains about "the
King" and how she's made use of him with the children.

The King, she says, is a loud, stern, blustering
character who visits the children in the classrooms,
crowns them and honors them, dubs them this or
that, and gives them simple commands like stand,
sit, or kneel. (He is only one of several characters
Janine has created, costumed, and made up for

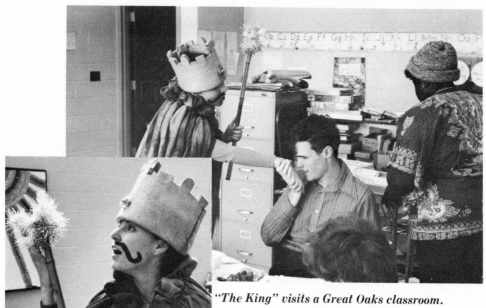

"The King" visits a Great Oaks classroom.
Janine Stone as "The King."

classroom appearances; there is also a Tree Creature and a Mouse and a Monster.) After she has demonstrated how the King moves and behaves, she gives the children a chance to get dressed up in the King's costume and play the role for themselves. Here are some of the responses she told me the King brought about that week:

Michael C. paraded through the halls to the office to show Lynn Johnson how he looked all dressed up as the King—moustache included. We couldn't find Lynn, but Michael knew who we were looking for and he craned his neck to check her office out. He was disappointed at not finding her, but he certainly enjoyed all the fuss people made over him.

Chrissy, who aloofly ignored direct attention and just lay near the window peeking out through the slits of her eyes—well, Chrissy was ordered on a "forced march of 10 miles" by the King, sternly and with lots of fanfare. Then I picked her up and march we did, and I kept bouncing her around roughly until she giggled with delight.

Before beginning the makeup and face paint-ing, I try to make the child aware of his or her face in the mirror–and the effect of applying color to accentuate facial parts. The greasepaint is heavy, and children are aware of it by feeling its pressure as well as by seeing it. The entire process is complicated, of course, by squiggling children and working around a 5-foot mirror.

Tammy responded well. She was confused at first and didn't like having her face touched. But when she really looked at herself in the mirror (and seemed to figure out that it was her—decorated) she was delighted and wanted more. She spent almost 20 minutes looking at herself in the mirror. She was anxious to see how the other kids looked but seemed to have no desire to show off her face to others. She did seem to vocalize more, too, as she became more comfortable with her looks.

Janine Stone (Drama)
Great Oaks Arts Team

A very exceptional incident occurred when Debbie in Room 111 (who is severely retarded and 'doesn't respond to any-thing') put on the crown and robe and, taking the scepter, paraded around her room and out into the halls. She was not only altering her normal gait to a slower, more majestic pace, but (it seemed to me) she was actually *playing* the role. Teach-ers stopped to watch her pass and people in the hall noticed a real radiance of personal energy. It was definitely a highlight of my work so far.

Janine believes that her own art form—drama—encompasses movement, rhythm, music, and visual elements as well, and she's often able to integrate them with dramatic play. She describes dramatic play simply as "having fun inside some fanciful situation, an incident that's sometimes so normal it's overlooked with these kids. We engage in make-believe. Not just pretend you're a king or a pussycat but—and I firmly believe this—pretend you can walk, pretend you can talk, pretend you're

Some interesting things are happening with the costumes and masks I bring into the rooms. Billy wore the bird's head and sunglasses and Keith was replete with moustache and beard. A kind of sword fight seemed to be taking place between them for a moment. . . . Billy loved wearing glasses and watching himself. He would giggle and play peek-a-boo with the box lid and provide lots of verbal response (at least it sounds *like language). . . . When Stevie sees a cape, of any kind, he now twirls around the room instead of walking. . . . And little 18-month-old Michael F. reached up and pulled the beak off my bird mask yesterday; he seemed very interested in it even though, according to Fran, his teacher, he knew it wasn't his bottle.*

One failure: Maggie went from only having seizures when I tried to work with her to seizing every time she saw me!

Janine Stone (Drama)
Great Oaks Arts Team

---

the boss of the world, pretend you don't have to sit inside all your life."

Janine's repertoire of dramatic activities with the children embraces other kinds of dramatic play, and often draws on other art forms as well. Among those she found to be effective:

• Hiding behind fanciful masks and playing peek-a-boo

• Using makeup to paint the children's faces in front of large mirrors so they can see how they look

• Making up rhyming-name poems to encourage vocalization, even for deaf-blind children like "Willie Crete" who comes close and feels her breath on his face ("Willie Crete, Sweet Treat, You're Neat Enough to Eat")

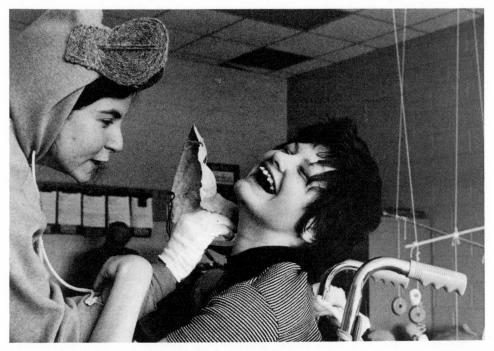

Janine, in Mouse costume, nibbles Tammie's neck.

• Calling on her full-dress Mouse character to play Hickory Dickory Dock up and down the children's bodies, mainly those who are seriously involved

• Playing Hey Diddle Diddle accompanied by the percussion sounds of a tambourine ("Brian, who has some hearing, was delighted with the sounds and responded with a soft hum, which I encouraged by mirroring the sound")

• Using the puppets the teachers have in their rooms to create a host of fanciful dramatic situations

Janine, despite her bias toward her chosen art form, thinks it's the artist not the art form as such that's essential to this kind of work. "You can go to art school or drama school," she contends, "and graduate with honors but that doesn't necessarily mean you come out an artist. An artist simply feels, senses, looks at the world in a particular way . . . and I'm convinced it's the kind of *people* we are, not what we *do*, that makes it work here, with these kids."

In one of the classrooms up on the second floor I find the music person on the Great Oaks team, Michele Valeri. Michele is a slim, dark-haired young woman in blue jeans who's seated at a table among a group of children and their two teachers. She's singing "She'll Be Comin' Round the Mountain!" and accompanying herself on a guitar. The children are all in the profound category and, in chronological age, somewhere in their teens. Some pay no attention to Michele, but most seem to be joining in; others—with encouragement from her or the teachers—manage a few sounds.

She leads them in "Oh! Susanna" and several other such repetitive folk songs and then she abruptly shifts gears. Distributing various kinds of rhythm instruments—a tin drum, a cabasa, vibes, a shaker, a tambourine, and two corrugated cardboard blocks that can be rubbed together to make washboard sounds—she begins another kind of song in which, at appropriate places, the children are encouraged to strike, shake, rattle, or stroke their respective instruments. The song is called "Are You My Mother?" a question asked of each child in turn by a small hand puppet named Fred who's operated now by one of the teachers.

When it's his turn to respond, nearly every child needs to be specifically cued several times as well ("Okay, Paul—hit the drum!"). And this indeed is the ultimate purpose—to make use of a song in which tempo, pauses, and repetitive-action verses all call for a specific gross-motor action in response to a verbal cue (spoken or sung). Here, too, the puppet who is searching for his mother adds a dramatic element and provides a character for the children to relate to more personally.

What Artists Can Bring To SPH Kids

The artist is there to be vulnerable. You can't be an artist unless you expose yourself to whatever life has to offer—and this kind of work exposes you right down to the raw.

Because—you're being asked to love (or like at least) what is generally regarded as unlovable. You're asked to reach out and touch the lives of those we've tried to put out of sight, to avoid, because we don't want to deal with what they represent. In this sense, you're being asked to celebrate with the living dead.

The contribution you, as artists, are making here is partly this: because of what you are and what you are able to give of yourself, you have a unique capacity to block out all the visible trappings of what these children are and reach deep into the human being trapped inside.

You've selected your own art form because of what you are. And you're going to use it to see if, somehow, we can turn this human situation around . . . to inch it on to whatever percentage more it can be! What it might really become, for any given child who rides out there on your artistry, is just awesome!

George Latshaw

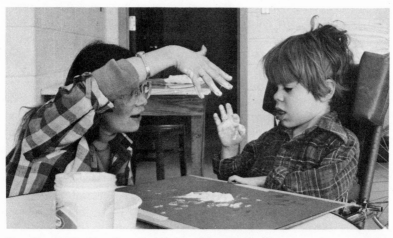

Pam Lowenthal teaches Andy a hand-to-mouth response using a marshmallow substance as art material.

I realize that the teachers need to be worked with as much as the children. Though most of them are strong and caring, their morales are delicate. It can be depressing work, and I believe they need to be joining in with the music activities as much as the children do.

I find myself relating to them during the lessons, with asides and questions as I go along, because I really do need their support. The situation here involves mutual assistance— which may seem obvious but isn't always. I realize I'm there basically to be adding to their program, to be helping them. But in approaching it with the very real awareness of how much of their help I need, I've seen how the teachers' attitudes can make the class work for you, and the lesson work for the children.

Michele Valeri (Music)
Great Oaks Arts Team

Afterwards, Michele explains to me that this was the first time the entire class stayed seated at the table for a full half hour:

The fact that no one wandered off was a source of pride to me. Mary, the aide, told me she thought they really enjoyed it. Curtis threw the tambourine a few times and Stevie couldn't rub the washboards, but he did hit one against the other. Next time I'll give him the same instrument and see what happens. Michael actually reached for the vibes with the mallet, too, and plunked a few notes with Mary's help.

It's fascinating about the puppet. Michael loved Fred, so did Paul. They all acknowledged his presence, except maybe Curtis—I couldn't tell about him. Stevie didn't like Fred so he ignored him, but he did know he was there and asking something, I'm sure. I felt it was one of my best classes, not because the children did anything spectacular but because they *attended* the whole time. I felt they were "all there," except at times I could feel myself losing Curtis.

Michele has a theater background (principally in creative dramatics) as well as a talent for vocal and

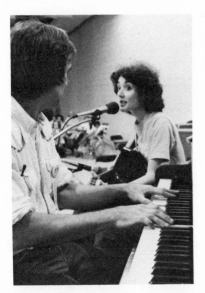

Michele Valeri singing to Latshaw puppet (above piano) at Great Oaks VSAF.

The therapist suggested I sit on the right side of Michael because he has reflexive muscle spasms that keep him leaning to the left. He's blind, but he loves the sound of the mandolin. So we propped him up with his head cushioned so it would remain straight ahead—and I took his left hand and brought it across his body to where the mandolin was. At first he stiffened and then, more relaxed, he began strumming the strings. The therapist was very pleased at this. We played "Zippidee-Do-Dah" and Michael strummed away pretty happily for quite awhile.

This was the first time I have worked with just one student, and I see the value in the "one-on-one" interaction. Group activities are fine but there has to be a balance between those things and the kinds of things I can do with children individually.

Michele Valeri (Music)
Great Oaks Arts Team

instrumental music. She also composes some of the songs she sings as an entertainer in Washington-area clubs—and she tells me she's beginning to make up songs about a few of the children here. They're mostly songs in which the words and the rhythm emphasize some action that teachers have mentioned are among the objectives they've set for a particular child. There's a song she's called "Put Your Finger in the Air" about yet another boy named Michael who needs to keep his fingers flexing rather constantly and a song called "Ankles" about a 9-year-old black boy named Antonio who has to wear leg braces. (See Appendix for a case study on Antonio)

Music appears to be an art form that has an unusually broad application for the severely and profoundly handicapped population. Obviously there is a deep measure of sheer enjoyment that can be generated among the higher functioning children whenever familiar tunes are played or sung, when

One day I went in to Eileen's room and after we did the "band sound" activity, she said, "You know, Reggie can sing. He's learned 'Comin' Round the Mountain.'" Reggie's a large, profoundly retarded black boy of 18. Well—I started that song and then I stopped, and Eileen said, "C'mon, Reggie, it's your turn." And it was like that music came from way far inside of him, but he worked at it and worked at it and finally did it twice all the way through— kind of husky and soft. It was wonderful—and I'm going to get him to learn some more of those folk songs.

Michele Valeri (Music)
Great Oaks Arts Team

they sing as part of a group or get to make sounds with the various stringed or rhythm instruments. But music lends itself to work with the more seriously involved children as well—when it can cue a specific physical or verbal response, emphasize a body part or an action, and provide teachers with fresh ways to bring about a response or to work on a specific objective.

It takes patience, alertness, and considerable trial and error, as Michele points out, to discover the key to a particular child's psyche, to find out what will best motivate him and unlock his response in some way, indeed to learn what *not* to do with him, and even to recognize behaviors that don't mean what they *seem* to mean.

She explains how little 8-year-old Brian, who's in "the baby's room down the hill", gave her (with the help of an aide) one kind of clue:

When I first went in there, the aide said she didn't think much would happen with those kids because they don't move or do anything much. They sleep most of the time. But I kept bringing in my instruments and finally got them strumming them, and they seemed to like that. But then one day I brought in my guitar and played it with Brian, and he began to cry. I wanted to stop because I thought it was making him feel bad for some reason, but the aide said, "No, keep going. He's not pulling away!" So, in this case, I learned that crying isn't the message; the crying is something else, and it has nothing to do with what I'm doing. The message was the *pulling back* was the thing to look for . . . and now I know that with Brian.

At noon Michele and Janine depart. The following morning the two other members of the team—Graceanne Adamo and Pam Lowenthal—appear for the first of their two weekly visits of 3 hours each. Graceanne is a professional dancer and dance teacher who has just opened her own dance studio in Bethesda. Pam is a visual artist who has a university degree in fine arts and is now working on her master's in art therapy; she is, incidentally, the only member of the Great Oaks group who has had some previous experience working with SPH kids.

Graceanne believes the unique contributions of dance to this project lie in providing an opportunity for both the ambulatory *and* the nonambulatory children to move and be moved *simply for movement's sake*. "The nonambulatory kids are moved to be cleaned, to breathe more easily, or to be placed where they can sleep—but not much else. By the end of our project I hope it'll be the norm around here for teachers, aides, and artists to scoop up a nonambulatory child and dance with him." (At least one teacher took exception to this, by the way; "it was *already* the norm for teachers to dance with nonambulatory kids," she reported to me later. "In fact, we were doing many of these things before the artists came in.")

The ambulatory children, Graceanne says, are almost all in the Behavior-Management classes. A great part of what they are learning, of course, is to respond appropriately to situations and directions. Graceanne tells me:

When they dance with me, their teachers, or with the entire class, there's an opportunity for a positive experience in a de-

"There Is Response —And It Is Expressive!"

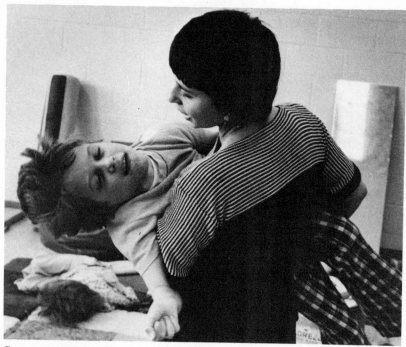

Graceanne Adamo dancing with Billy.

We each approach the problem in our own disparate yet related ways. Janine is very verbal and prop-oriented, Pam is materials-oriented, Michele is audience-involvement-in-live-music-oriented and I'm kinesthetically oriented. Although

manding social situation requiring concentrated and close physical action—with a relative stranger (me) and with other people they know well. I've begun to feel that many of these children who are exploring space more daringly with their bodies are starting to associate movement with a kind of plea-

we felt some responsibility to develop things uniquely, we've tried more and more to integrate our forms and approaches and to get a true sense of what would be involved in an inter-arts approach.

You learn that these kids won't readily tolerate the lesson plans, rationale descriptions, or graded activities of regular schooling. They don't care who you know or where you've performed or what you are wearing. In that sense, working with them is somewhat akin to performing; when you're on stage, whatever happens is all that exists.

The SPH child is an existentialist. He lives in the now. He will seldom be able to tell you what happened last week, or why he won't talk or walk, or why he has little sense of what's going to happen tomorrow. He is as he is in this moment. If you are to be with him, you must share that moment. I see this, really, as the unique relationship that can be established between the artist and the SPH child.

I know that the more I can get a child to do with me, the better I can come to know and understand him . . . to sense the multidimensional nature of his existence, not merely his appearance or the regular sounds he makes. I feel more at ease with the ambulatory kids, but the nonmovers are the more challenging because the only thing that happens with them is what I can make happen.

The responses of these children to those around them and to the arts situations could not be called less than expressive. For some it probably is the most expressive they've ever been. Much of this expressiveness, of course, would have no interest for an audience of the general public. But it is very important communication for those around them who deal with the child. Whether the child is tolerating, wildly enjoying, or even ignoring the activity—there is response and it is expressive.

Graceanne Adamo (Dance)
Great Oaks Arts Team

sure and success that's quite unlike what they get from putting together a wooden puzzle successfully.

Graceanne's activities obviously rely heavily on music; sometimes she teams up with Michele for this, but mainly the bouncy, cheerful pop music she uses is provided by records that she brings into the classrooms. In one classroom the music is on as I enter, and she's working with a group of ambulatory children, helping them master a simple movement: they are holding on to her hand as they run in a circle and getting used to leaning their bodies away from center.

One little boy is capable of running apparently, but he resists hand contact. So Graceanne decides to run alone and encourage him to join her; but it doesn't work—he seems unable or unwilling to imitate her. Next she tries jumping, but he won't imitate that action either. Finally she uses a technique which (she tells me later) she'd observed a teacher doing: she stands behind the child and lifts him off the floor in a series of jumping actions. He begins laughing, obviously enjoying this, so she uses it in what she calls an "antecedent-consequence" manner; she simply runs awhile and then jumps, runs awhile and then jumps. Soon he's doing what she wanted him to do originally.

Trial and error. Patience. Alert observation. And inventiveness. Meanwhile the music has stopped, the turntable is dulling the needle, and Graceanne realizes that soon she must go on to the next room without getting to work individually with several of the other children in this room today. Part of the penalty involved in this sort of slow, patient individualized work.

I learn that earlier she has introduced a striking new phenomenon into the school environment, a "Dancing Snake" that she's used to generate all kinds of responses. The Snake is a ready-made toy, actually—a tube tunnel made of rubberized material about 10 feet long that's supported by wire rounds. What happens is this:

Graceanne enters each room wearing the Snake over her vertically, as a cylinder that covers her from head to foot. She carries several instruments over her shoulders *inside* the cylinder—drum, tambourine, bells—which she now begins playing. The music makes the snake undulate, rotate, and lean ponderously over the children. As she approaches the children, she enfolds them in the cylinder, allowing them to touch it, push it, move it along with her inside it. (The soft rubber material covering the Snake is ventilated with pinholes that allow the person in it to see out but not be seen.)

The ambulatory children are soon putting it over them, as she has done, and are walking around with it on. When it's placed horizontally on the floor many children crawl or scoot through it. Some of the children like the feeling of insulated security so much they have to be coaxed to come out—only to dive back in. Some found that, while they were inside they could also roll it along the floor.

Graceanne described several of the more enchanting reactions:

Reggie became ecstatic over the whole thing. He tried to peer into the top to discover what was inside. When he found it was me in there, he jumped up and down with delight. When I lowered the top end so he could put it over his head and share being in there with me, he held both of my hands and danced around with the Snake. Holly was a little intimidated at first but definitely interested. She has trouble with new things but, with some coaxing, Angie [her teacher] got her to scoot through it on her bottom.

In Billy's room Michele was there at the same time and, while she played the guitar and sang, the Snake gyrated vigorously. Billy, who was out of his wheelchair and lying on a mat, was apparently moved enough by all this to play—repeatedly, with obvious intention and control—a toy organ which Michele had placed on the mat next to him.

Graceanne believes the big outsized nature of the Snake truly fascinates all the children. It helps overcome fears and, at the same time, provides a sense of security. She thinks that, although it's a movement device that obviously works best with ambulatory children, it does seem to generate favorable responses in the nonambulatory kids as well—especially when teachers can manipulate it to enclose the kids where they sit, or lie, or stand in their "standing" chairs. It's also fun for many of those kids simply to watch the Snake as it moves around in space.

Pam Lowenthal's specialty is the visual arts. For work with this population, one would expect it to be a more circumscribed art form since the visual arts don't involve the sheer physicality of the performing arts—the lively, uninhibited movement, the dramatic play, the tantalizing sounds and rhythmic music. Lacking those elements that can induce broader kinds of physical and vocal action among more able kids, the visual arts also pose problems for the more seriously involved children who may not have the fine motor skills required to manipulate the artist's materials. Furthermore, it is difficult to work with such materials in large groups and maintain any effective instructional control. And it's apt to be messy too; in spite of any covering you provide them, the kids will find ways to smear themselves with (and/or eat) the paint, glue, plaster, clay, and especially the chocolate pudding you use for finger painting.

Pam Lowenthal readily acknowledges these matters but doesn't seem at all inhibited by them. She simply takes her work in a different direction, using arts activities she already knows about or inventing new ones to meet the SPH kids' special situations. She depends on such activities as body tracing, finger painting (using foodstuffs), making plaster shapes, wrapping bodies in colored tissue paper (in front of a large mirror and then showing the kids how they look), and making sculptures by gluing variously shaped wooden blocks together.

Most of these approaches, she has found, are applicable to both low- and high-functioning kids. The glued-block sculptures, on the other hand, along with such traditional art activities as drawing and painting, making "sandtable" landscapes and cities, and working more skillfully in clay or plaster, Pam

uses regularly with the older, less physically disabled youngsters (and often, she says proudly, "with
great success").

Her observations about some of these activities
suggest why the visual arts can hold their own with
the performing arts in this work:

• *Colored Tissue Paper and Mirror.* This business of
wrapping the kids in colored tissue paper is effective
both with sighted kids [who react to the colors] and
with blind kids [who can hear it crackle when you
crumple it up and then get tactile stimulation from
its rough texture].... Holly allowed me to tape
many colors on her, around the arms, legs, and
torso—with the final touch being a triangle over her
head like a scarf. She sat in front of the mirror for 20
minutes (maybe longer, as I left her that way) and
stared at herself, touching the mirror every so often
with her hands.... Billie loved having the paper
scarf around his head—he usually doesn't like having you touch him near his face. Maybe it was the
sound it made. Anyway, he smiled and giggled and
made lots of vowel sounds and "yes" sounds when I
patted the paper over his ear.... Andy, who usually
screams when touched, didn't seem to mind being
covered—and then he sat and watched me cover the
others....

• *Body Tracing.* For more able and mobile children,
body tracing was pretty successful.... Judy, profoundly retarded and aged 16 in Room 9, "attended"
to the tracing process with some enjoyment, I
thought—and very little rocking or head throwing,
especially when I drew her face in for her. She identified her shoe on the tracing, too!... Phelicia, in
Louise's room, also liked seeing her facial features
drawn in—and she tried to color them herself!...
When somebody tore up Chucky's tracing, he was
very upset and came down to the office for more
paper so he could do another one.... Karen,

"I Had To Tap Way Down To The Basics of Expression"

My involvement in this project has increased my creative thinking, because I had to tap way down to the basics of expression in order to find ways of offering art to these children. Rather than relying on skill, talent, or style, I began to rely more on basic thoughts, responses, and experiences. I opened my eyes more to what children do every day—how normal children begin to experience things that can become art (banging pans together, spreading food with their fingers, etc.).

I think probably the visual arts have the most effect on these kids' physical development, affective development, and social development—in that order. Physically, the child can learn grasping, pointing, squeezing (to develop muscles), pulling, waving arms—all of which are used when drawing, tearing paper, or working with clay.

When a child's trying to work with different materials, there are all kinds of emotions coming to the surface—happiness, disgust, excitement, frustration. You can actually see the child's reaction to different substances, and you can watch their expressions when they see that they can make something happen when they hold a wet brush and move it across a paper with felt-pen colors on it.

And socially, it seems to me they learn to respond to one another's artistic work. They become more intrigued with what each of them does—and the higher functioning children can actually begin to fantasize, using their own creations, and communicate on new levels with one another.

Elmer, in Marlene's room, likes to be physically close. As long as I was next to him, he would draw pretty contentedly. Once, when the children were working on a mural placed on the floor, he scooted over next to me when I moved away from him. It seemed to give him a sense of security—and also assured him of my immediate attention!

Pam Lowenthal (Visual Art)
Great Oaks Arts Team

Chucky, and John F. in Phyllis's room all loved the experience and worked very hard and carefully coloring their outlines. Karen asked me to do a second one with her. . . . I plan to follow this up by having these higher functioning kids trace each other, and then see if they can draw faces and body parts that aren't tracings.

• *Wooden Block Sculptures.* I brought in some small wooden blocks of different shapes and some glue and showed the kids in Marlene's room how to brush on the glue and stick the blocks together. There was a pretty good response to this complicated task. . . . Elmer seemed to understand that the flat side of wood had to be glued to another flat piece, not a rounded side. . . . When we did it again two weeks later, Elmer wanted to show his special friend—a former teacher who had come back to visit—what he'd done, and he remembered the whole process. He glued *three* pieces together to build a tower, and kept looking to his teacher for praise. They *all* seemed to remember what to do and every kid produced at least one block sculpture—with a little assistance from me to keep them from eating the glue. . . . I'm going to keep all the finished pieces and bring them in again later—with a large sheet of heavy cardboard so we can build a city.

• *Felt Pens, Water, Brush, and White Paper.* This painting activity has produced some interesting responses. I usually demonstrate it first. . . . with the felt pen. I'll scribble colors on large white paper that's taped to a board and placed in front of each kid, either on a table or against the wall; I'll wet the brush and put it in a child's hand, helping him move the brush over the colors. It's great to watch the children respond to the color changes, the blendings and drippings—and then most of them want to do it themselves. . . . Stevie, the profoundly handicapped 21-year-old boy in Louise's room, was lying in a corner on a mat, but when I said, "Let's draw a picture, Stevie." He got up right away, went to the table, and began using the pens and brushes. He was also able to copy a circle when I demonstrated it. . . . Michael W. in Cathy's room—he's 14 and profoundly retarded—responded with real enthusiasm and great effort. He tries hard to control his arms which flail about in spasms (often he just weighs one hand down with the other), but he seems to enjoy making marks and colors on *large* spaces—it's more frustrating for him, obviously, when he's confined to a space requiring more control. . . . Eugenia watches the colors change and dissolve and doesn't get as upset as usual. . . . Andy wouldn't take the brush in hand but watched with fascination when others created new color blendings with the brush and water.

What seems to characterize the artists on this Great Oaks team more than anything else, perhaps, is their style. Whatever their off-project manners and demeanors may have been, their impact on the Great Oaks environment seemed imbued with extraordinary personal style. Each of them had it (Pam, the *non*performing artist of the bunch, included) and while they each exhibited it somewhat differently, the basic ingredients were much the same.

They almost always seemed to be bringing verve and dash and spontaneity to their tasks. Full of energy, often boisterous (and sometimes even a bit unruly) they would arrive spiritedly on the scene and burst in on classrooms almost as though they'd geared themselves up to "take stage" (as performers put it) during their entire 3-hour visits. Their teaching styles almost precisely embodied the attributes that George Latshaw believes equip the artist, almost uniquely, for effective work with these children: a willingness to place oneself at risk, a personal inventiveness and resourcefulness, and a readiness to try just about anything and, if it doesn't work, to try something else. These artists also possessed a kind of exposed vulnerability that comes from not keeping a constant guard on one's feelings.

Here and there among the teachers, to be sure, some of this may well have seemed more like excessive "artistic temperament." Yet, if this could be said to represent a modest minority viewpoint of the teachers in all three sites, there was still a solid majority who valued—or *learned* to value—these mercurial characteristics highly. As one teacher observed:

"It seems to me that the artist's special contributions had a great deal to do with their uninhibited manner and personalities. The nice thing about them was that they showed us it was okay to goof around, do crazy things, make fools of themselves."

Stephanie Mance, a Great Oaks teacher, put it this way: "In our personal lives, or in our everyday interactions with our peers, we may tend to be more inhibited than we would with the kids in the classroom. Lack of inhibition is what is most effective in getting a response from the kids—doing whatever you have to do to get a reaction. And the artists really supported that idea through their uninhibited behavior and presentations in the classroom."

Seventeen individual artists were engaged to work on the project during the pilot period; three were replaced early on, however, and the working number remained at fourteen throughout. All but one, Doug Genschmer, the visual arts person on the Walton team (plus one of those replaced), were women. They had all obtained their undergraduate degrees, some in the arts, but, interestingly enough, the greater number majored in arts education, arts therapy, or special education. Some had received their master's degrees, as well, in these same general fields, and perhaps half a dozen, in the Dallas and Stockton sites especially, were currently enrolled in graduate programs.

Each team was made up of representatives of the four major art forms—music, dance, drama, and the visual arts. In Stockton, these team members were all recruited from among the instructional staff at the Alan Short Center, the cultural arts institution offering arts classes and experiences to moderately handicapped adults. Somewhat in contrast to the Great Oaks team members, they seemed to be directing their professional lives and ambitions more toward careers as arts teachers and arts therapists than toward professional studio work and performance.

Doug Genschmer, the visual arts person, had obtained art education degrees in Iowa and had taught art in regular public schools and in an institution for retarded children. The three other members of the Stockton team, interestingly enough, all had some experience in the music therapy field—but two appeared to be generalists enough, as well, to take on project responsibility in art forms other than those in which they'd received professional training.

Debi Ross had graduated from University of the Pacific a year earlier as a registered music therapist and managed to combine that with a performance degree in flute; since then, she'd been teaching at the Alan Short Center, giving private flute lessons, taking creative movement classes at the university, and performing with local bands and choirs. Her responsibility at Walton was dance, however, a field she had bridged into somewhat from music—via folk dancing, and square dancing in particular.

Maria Rubino, engaged as the Stockton team's drama person, also had a music therapy background and had taken work under Claudine Sherrill at Texas Woman's University. Her dramatic interests had been developed through performance experiences with amateur little theatre groups, chiefly in children's theater. Celeste Behnke, also deeply involved in music and music therapy during her undergraduate years, was the team member actually hired as the music specialist. She had recently enrolled in a graduate program in special education at UC-Sacramento and had come to the Alan Short

Center that fall to begin 6 months of music therapy internship.

In Dallas, the standard four-person team had been expanded to six. In order to work around the off-project schedules of some team members, Randy Routon, the site team leader, had assigned two people (Vickie Moore and Barbara Baxley) to conduct the music activities jointly and two others (Rosie Gonzales and Carol Kay Harsell) to share the dance position on the SCS team.

Like those on the Walton Team, most of these young women seemed to be moving toward careers in arts education, adapted recreation, or arts therapy of some kind, and were currently pursuing advanced degrees at TWU. Most were also involved in part-time work with handicapped populations under the several BEH and NCAH projects that Claudine Sherrill was directing. The exception was Barbara Baxley, who had taken her undergraduate work at North Texas State and was a registered music therapist with a recently completed master's degree from Southern Methodist University.

Darlene Seguin, the visual arts person, was an arts educator who'd taught in south Texas schools and first worked with retarded children when she came to Dallas a few years earlier to take a job in the city recreation department. Wishing to enter the field of art therapy, she too was working toward a master's at TWU, one that combined art education and special education.

Carol Kay Harsell's background included a period when she danced professionally; however, during the project only Vickie Moore and the Dallas team's drama person, Kathy Burks, appeared to be active professionally as artists—rather than as arts educators or arts therapists. Vickie Moore was keeping her hand in professionally by working as a pianist in summer musical theaters in Missouri. Kathy Burks, with a background in puppetry and music, was

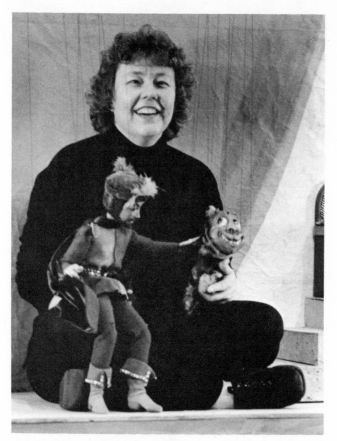

Kathy Burks with characters from her marionette play.

directing a resident marionette theater, The Haymarket Theatre Company, in a unique north Dallas shopping center. The company develops and produces original children's theater works, mostly tailored to the 1,000-odd characters of the famed Sue Hastings Marionettes which Kathy inherited some years ago. The group also stages live theater productions for adult audiences in the evenings. Kathy was the only project drama person, incidentally, whose experience was extensive enough in puppetry to give professional follow-up to the Latshaw workshops.

Special Care School, March 1979

Around noon, the big orange Dallas school bus turns into the Special Care School parking area and draws up outside the building. It's lunch time at SCS, but the students are too excited to care much about eating. Although most of these children live almost entirely in the present and have little awareness of what the future (remote or immediate) holds, they seem to sense that something special is in the offing this afternoon. Something is going to happen: somehow, instinctively, they feel it.

And indeed they are right. When lunch is over, the entire student body, the teachers, and aides will climb aboard the bus and venture forth on what will be the first of several project-related field trips scheduled for the weeks ahead.

Unlike Walton or Great Oaks, SCS is not a "busing school." The kids are transported to and from school by their parents, so simply boarding a huge school bus, getting settled down in the seats, and riding off in it—whatever the destination—is an experience in itself. Clearly, something of this impending adventure has already communicated itself to the students; Roger and I, in fact, have timed our second visit to SCS to coincide with this particular event.

We suspect, however, that if all the children fully comprehended where the bus would be taking them today, the excitement might be even more unbridled, for this is a field trip to the theater. The busload of SCS kids will travel across town to the Ollapodrida Shopping Center, where Kathy Burks's Haymarket Theatre is located, for a special performance of a marionette play written and produced by Kathy's company. All of us can hardly wait.

Since our arrival, earlier in the week, we've been reorienting ourselves to the special qualities of this Special Care School. We've had a chance to move in and out of the classrooms, as always; to reestablish relationships with the children—with Lori and Raymond and Glen and Stuart and Catherine and the others—and to renew acquaintances with their teachers. And of course there have been opportunities to catch up with what the arts team has been doing since our initial visit.

Because the Special Care School is smaller and less complex than the other sites, the reorientation process doesn't take very long; the openness and friendliness that is characteristic here (in Texas?) has soon enveloped us again.

With the arts team, I am on the lookout for similarities (and differences) of approach with respect to the other sites. And not unsurprisingly, there's a little of both in the way this SCS team goes about things.

The similarities are readily apparent. They resort to many of the same kinds of arts activities (songs, games, movements); they bring in some of the same kinds of materials to work with (paper, paints, costumes); and they use many of the same kinds of instruments, equipment, and props.

There's really no overall quality about the artists that stands out, however, as a singular characteristic — as *style* does in the Great Oaks team. These six women artists are a mixture of personal qualities. Several bring a kind of irrepressible enthusiasm to their work with children — a zest and a lilt that are contagious. Others have a steady reassuring quality about them; more thoughtful, perhaps, they move among the children with a quiet, friendly patience that's most persuasive.

Their purpose is to reach and motivate these special children and, whatever their manner of approach may be, these artists stay with it—seeking for the things that work best with each child. They are inventive, too, each in her own way, and they all seem to have planned the things they are doing with considerable care and forethought.

They have, from the beginning, gone about their

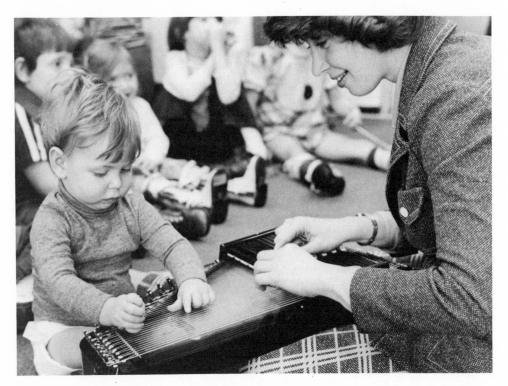

Barbara Baxley helps Corey to "play" the autoharp.

These SPH kids are much like very young normal children who "make music" by beating the drum or a xylophone. They don't have any real sense of music **per se** *because they're not able to comprehend the organization of sound and silence in music. A child like this simply makes "noise" and, although the sounds may be pleasant, they aren't music. He does have the satisfaction of "playing" the instrument, however, . . . he's produced the sound* **himself.** *He's involved in the [music-making] process at his own level of functioning. Even very seriously involved children almost always respond with some form of eye contact to the sound of any instrument–or to singing–and they'll often reach out and try to touch the source of the sound.*

Barbara Baxley (Music)
SCS Arts Team

The children at SCS taught me more than I could have ever hoped to teach them. The word "creativity" has a completely new meaning to me now. You learn that there are as many ways to use music as there are people in the world. You just have to be that flexible. You have to shape the environment—and then be ready to work with any kind of response that occurs!

Vickie Moore (Music)
SCS Arts Team

---

work more as educators would—something that derives clearly from the training that many of them are involved in with Claudine Sherrill at Texas Woman's University. For the most part, each team member has been encouraged to become familiar with the children's individual educational plans— the IEPs—and several even went so far as to build an IEP card file that listed each child's teacher-developed goals on one side and, on the other, a group of arts activities they felt had potential for helping to realize these goals.

Barbara Baxley (who, with Vickie Moore, is responsible for music activities here) tells me that "knowing the IEP goals saved me hours and *weeks* of trial and error experimentation, of trying to figure out for myself the functional level of each child and what direction to go in with him." (There is another side to this IEP matter, of course, and the pros and cons—centering ultimately on whether team members regard themselves more as artists or as teachers—is delineated more fully on pages 112–115).

Similarities and differences aside, however, some of my early impressions about members of this SCS team emerge once again during this second visit and are reinforced. For instance, Barbara and Vickie seem, during their music sessions, to have a special fondness for instruments like the xylophone and the autoharp (and even for a set of "jingle bells" which they've found helps to motivate response in some of the children). Certainly, they're easier than the traditional stringed instruments (guitar, banjo, mandolin) to get the kids to manipulate, to "make music" on—and both women encourage a good deal of this when they work individually with each child.

Barbara points out that almost every young child will beat on a drum or bang on a piano—and that these sounds aren't really music, they're just "noise." But they're sounds he's produced himself and, in his way, he's actually "played" the instrument (see box p. 85).

Like their counterparts elsewhere, Barbara and Vickie depend heavily on *singing* activities of all kinds, regardless of the degree of handicap characterizing the class. There's not a great deal of singing *to* or playing music *for* the children, except in the case of those who have little movement. The idea is to get each child to participate in some way, so most of the singing is built around group activities, to stimulate sing-along responses or to produce a vocal or eye-contact response from an individual child.

Barbara and Vickie's repertoire for these occasions consists of many melodies that one associates with childhood or nursery rhymes, but there are plenty of the campfire variety as well—catchy tunes, old songfest standbys, folksongs, and the special songs they make up themselves. One of the most effective uses of this kind of tune, they have found, is to adapt it to the teaching of proper names and body parts—and it's not unusual to enter a classroom and hear, for instance, that "Lori's comin' round the mountain with her *nose*" (arm, leg, ear), or some such nonsensical creation. (Then: "Where *is* your nose, Lori? Can you find it for me?")

There are "hello" songs and "goodbye" songs too (sung to melodies like "Goodnight, Ladies"), and the music people make a specific point of directing these songs to each child individually, going around the room at the beginning and the end of class and singing with every child, one at a time.

This project has presented me with the greatest challenge I have ever had. It was my first encounter on a one-to-one basis with special children. It was a beautiful encounter. My personal creativity and aesthetic sense were reinforced tremendously. I am convinced the medium of the arts provides a special way to communicate with the special child. The joy of "just being" is somehow capsuled in this communication. The arts demand feelings, not always words. Because of this freedom I have found a much greater understanding and response from the children with whom I have been involved.

Kathy Burks (Drama)
SCS Arts Team

Rosie Gonzales and Carol Kay Harsell, who share responsibility for the dance classes, have been able to go beyond the point of movement for its own sake. Probably because a greater proportion of these SCS children are functioning at higher levels than at other sites, it's been possible for them to place more of an emphasis on some of the fundamentals of movement and even on the creative aspects of dance as an art form.

Both Carol Kay and Rosie conduct their dance sessions in the SCS gymnasium. At first, they tell me, the teachers would bring their children to the gym and leave—but now I notice that the teachers are not only remaining to observe but are actively participating, along with Tim Morris (the recreation specialist) and Julie Russell (the physical therapist).

Carol Kay explains what's happened to produce this attitude change:

I began to realize pretty early that it was going to be tough to work on each child's objectives in the time I had available. I decided it was a matter of having to *demonstrate* to the teachers that it's possible to blend the academic or physical goals with the arts—so I urged the teachers and aides to stay and work with me when I had their children. Soon they began coming on their own, and coming dressed prepared to move. They're a

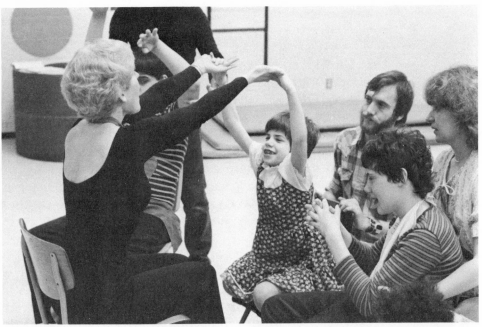

SCS children and teachers limber up in Carol Kay Harsell's dance-movement class.

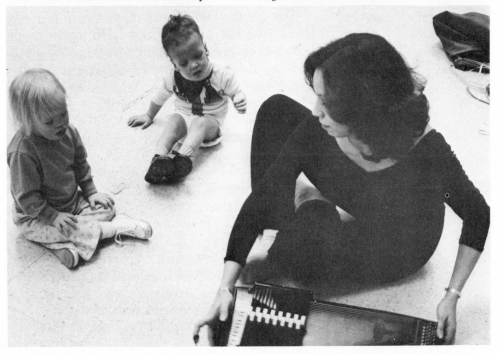

tremendous help, too, because they can control the rest of the class so I can work one-on-one with individuals, whenever there's time enough.

Carol Kay's classes, in fact, include many of the instructional elements one could observe in children's dance classes anywhere. She puts the children through a series of warm-up exercises at the beginning: stretching, bending, flexing, reaching, twisting—as the teachers and aides, sitting behind the children, help them follow her lead. (Following instructions, moving to a numbered count, large and small muscle activity, attending—these are some of the *nonarts* goals addressed, in this instance, by dance-movement.)

Then comes an opportunity for fanciful self-expression, as Carol Kay puts on a recording with a disco beat ("The Best of Earth, Wind and Fire") and encourages free-form improvised movement with scarves, streamers, balloons, and feathers as props. The nonambulatory kids take part as best they can, sitting or lying down. The others move around in the space in their own ways, and indeed Jimmy and one or two others reveal not only their uninhibited joy in the free-flowing movement itself but an unexpected imaginative quality that is lovely to watch as they weave and turn and bend to the music.

And then, as the period ends, Carol Kay changes the tempo of the recording, brings them back together, and instructs everybody to lie down on the floor and relax. This "quiet time," where there's a chance for the children to wind down and lie relatively still, next to their teachers, is an important part of the session; it sends them back to their academic classroom refreshed, loosened up, and diverted for a time—rather than hyperactive, overexcited, and hard to bring under what Hugh McBride, the Project's evaluator from University of the Pacific, has called "instructional control."

And Rosie reminds me that this control factor is just as essential for the arts team members as it is for the regular teachers, and it's a major reason for having the teachers present during the dance classes. "As Hugh says, we have to have the child under 'instructional control' before we can attempt to do much in the arts with him," she explains. "Otherwise we're spending half our time on behavior problems—and we're not trained for that."

They both make the distinction, however, between dance as therapy and dance as art. "My background in dance therapy has really helped me here," Carol Kay says. "But what I've been doing with the higher functioning kids is really 'Dance as an Art Form,' I'm convinced." And Rosie adds, "Anything you do for yourself that truly benefits you is therapy, I guess. So with the high-level kids, we do Dance (capital D) which has some therapeutic effects, and with the primary kids and some of the lower functioning kids, we're obviously doing therapy pure and simple, and movement is merely the medium we use to achieve our goals."

The things Darlene Seguin does in the visual arts seem to me to depend a bit more on the use of paints and clay than on such activities as cutting colored paper, working with wooden blocks, body tracing, or making costumes out of crumpled tissue paper—the things Pam Lowenthal works with a lot at Great Oaks. Darlene certainly doesn't exclude these things from her sessions (any more than Pam excludes work with paints and clay): in fact, one of Darlene's most successful activities is the imaginative one I find her engaged in with Glen and the other children in Sue Traghilla's Multiage Training Class.

She's taped a piece of white construction paper over a drum and covered the tips of some drumsticks with pieces of cloth. When they're dipped in paint, of course, they absorb it—and she's teaching the children to do this and then to "play the drum" with the colored drumsticks. For the lower functioning youngsters there is the simple enjoyment of banging

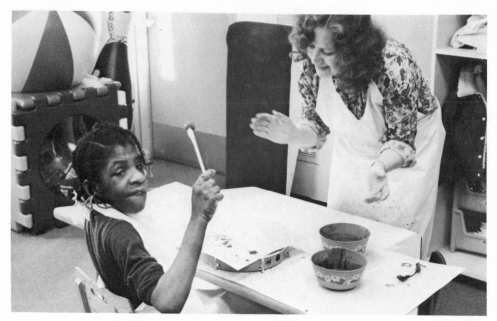

Darlene Seguin teaching Yolanda to "play the drum" with drumsticks dipped in paint.

noisily on the drum with something that leaves a mark, but it seems to go well beyond such random activity with some of the higher functioning children. "In the end," Sue points out later, "the paintings that resulted were really very unusual and some were beautifully done."

Darlene stresses to me that many of the abilities required for working with visual arts materials, of *any* kind, are also among the important *functional* and *cognitive* skills that the teachers are so purposefully training their children to acquire. There is, to be sure, in all the things one sees Darlene engaged in, a vast array of skills of this nature being called for: the kids are encouraged to do a lot of grasping, pinching, pushing, and pulling, along with activities that help with eye-hand coordination, shape and color identification, concentration and the lengthening of attention spans, or simply attending and following instructions. (This is a point I find echoed by the other visual artists, incidentally—by Pam Lowenthal at Great Oaks and Doug Genschmer at Walton—this extensive range of functional and cognitive skills which can be addressed by participation in the visual arts.)

Darlene notes something she (and the others as well) did *not* exactly expect would occur as an important outcome of this work. As she puts it, this has to do with the fact that "our visual art experiences are definitely influencing the children's social development. Obviously, it's because what we do encourages lots of interaction with the group. And it nearly always results in a finished product of some kind that acts as a catalyst for conversation in the class, something that can be held up and admired and shared with others."

This element of "socialization" turns out to be one of the more striking (and, for the teachers and some of the artists, unanticipated) outcomes of the project. There's little doubt that the drama is a major influence on this development—by its very nature, it forces social interaction. Certainly, too, the use of puppets by the drama people—and others as well—contribute strongly to such socialization outcomes, with Kathy Burks's professional background possibly giving the Special Care School a little advantage in this respect.

Finally, however, it is George Latshaw's continuing presence across the three project sites, his demonstrations, his puppet-making workshops for teachers and artists alike, his central philosophic approach, that make the drama-puppetry aspect of the project come alive. No matter in which school you find yourself, puppets and puppetry are increasingly in evidence among the teachers . . . a pervasive and delightful influence on all that is happening, artistically and educationally.

Even Kathy Burks isn't able to build in to her drama sessions very much that involves *marionettes* (puppets manipulated by strings from above rather than directly by hand), but her Haymarket Theatre offers the children a chance at least to see marionettes in an actual performance—and this particular field trip has been an obvious and long-awaited bonus from the beginning of the project.

But what ultimately is occurring here at the Haymarket Theatre this afternoon hasn't been anticipated by anyone—teachers, artists, or Kathy herself. In fact, the adult members of the audience can't quite believe what they now see taking place on the stage.

It's not the marionette play itself, which the company has just performed for the audience from SCS, although that has certainly been an entrancing and almost hypnotic experience for the children. To be sure, the play has produced its own amazements and surprises for the teachers: in spite of its length and complexity, it has held even those who are notoriously poor attenders enthralled and enrapt throughout.

The play is entitled *The Royal Enchantment* and is almost operettalike in form and style. It has been conceived and developed by the company here in part to make use of some of the famed Sue Hastings puppet collection. Based on a classical fairy story, it is the tale of a king and his beautiful daughter who come under the evil powers of a sorcerer who wants the kingdom for himself. The sorcerer turns the king into a walrus, his servant into a mouse—and himself into the king! The princess is banished to the far reaches of the kingdom with her walrus/father and a pair of enchanting baby tiger-cats she keeps on leashes. Ultimately, she and her father are saved by a brave young forester who outwits the sorcerer (by getting him to turn himself into a donkey by mistake). The sorcerer/donkey is duly banished in turn, the king is returned to his kingdom (and his own form), and the forester (of course) turns out to be a prince in disguise, and he and the princess fall in love and live happily ever after.

Much of this rather complicated narrative is told in song (over loudspeakers) and takes place in a series of very colorful settings. There are occasional hand-puppet characters operated from open trapped areas downstage, and the whole production is gloriously costumed and lighted in brilliant colors.

Enchanting as it is, however, the play runs almost a full hour, moves rather deliberately (and with long stretches of singing) from scene to scene, and has in it none of the Punch-and-Judy slapstick other such productions might have resorted to. In fact, Kathy Burks admits afterwards that she hasn't really been certain it was a production that would be appropriate for this particular audience, and she has even considered the possibility that it might well turn out to be a "total disaster."

Well, to the contrary, it has been an astounding success. This is not, to be sure, your customary well-behaved theater-going audience, and we have had our share of yips, shouts, and groans throughout the play—but looking back at the children's faces, from down front, I am confronted with almost total absorption: gleeful smiles, suspenseful anticipation, darting eyes following the action, intense concentration—and sheer delight in what's going on under the lights. The yips and shouts are their involuntary responses to the emotions engendered by the story.

And now, a different kind of delight and wonderment is being generated among the teachers, Roger and me, and Kathy and her fellow performers. The play has ended and the side and border drapes that form the proscenium opening have been drawn back to reveal the platform on which the people who operate the marionettes must stand. Kathy Burks's son, Doug, and her daughter, Becky, are on the platform manipulating several of the marionette figures we've just seen in the play.

For almost a half hour now, the children from SCS (those who are not confined to wheelchairs or who are not being held by adults) have been coming forward eagerly from their seats, climbing the steps to the stage and moving onto the set. Here, they've been playing and talking (interacting, the teachers call it) with the various marionette characters Doug and Becky have introduced from above and behind them.

Although there are occasional instances of kids jerking at the strings that control the marionettes, their response is remarkably free of the kind of excessive overreaction I at least had been half expecting. For the most part, it has been an orderly procession of children, moving up onto the stage, playing with the characters for a while (and particularly with the animal characters), and then moving back down to take their seats again and to watch as others take their place. Some of the teachers have been helping orchestrate all this, of course, while others have simply been sitting back and enjoying it, shaking their heads in amazement at the range and intensity of the children's interactions and responses.

Catherine, Glen, Ray, Rosie, Jimmy, Raymond (who couldn't help hamming it up to his friends in the house), Lori—*all* of them, in fact, have had us pointing, exclaiming, laughing (and almost crying) over their antics. Inevitably the animal characters (the walrus, the donkey, the mouse and, most of all, the two baby cats leaping about playfully) have triggered the most endearing responses. Wondrously touching and uproariously funny in turn, this magical moment has extended itself, as the kids poke, pat, and romp with the animals. Some, of course, aren't sure at first that they want to get too close, but (keeping a wary eye on the walrus especially) they too finally succumb.

What has captivated and astonished us all, though, is Stuart, a little 9-year-old with Down's syndrome in Joan Tyner's class (see the case study in the appendix page 154). On the border between severe and profound, Stuart (Joan has told us) often

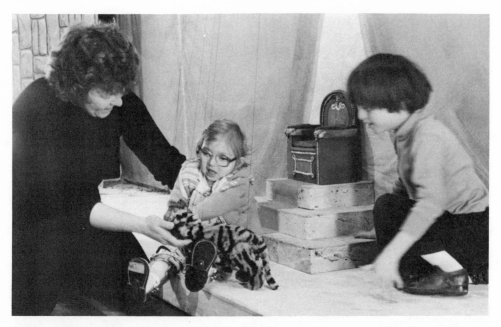

Kathy Burks on stage with Brandy and Stuart after marionette show.

uses puppets and other stuffed animals for self-stimulation purposes, rubbing or banging them against his teeth or his ear. And his attention span is seldom very lengthy.

But Stuart has been up on the stage the whole time. For over a half hour now, as the other children have come and gone, he has been totally absorbed in the marionette people and animals, and there has been hardly a moment when he's indulged in self-stimulation. He's virtually oblivious to everything going on around him.

The two baby cats and the donkey are his favorites. Mostly he sits on the edge of a little platform hugging and stroking and nuzzling them, talking quietly to them, or sometimes just gazing at them intently, face to face. Joan tells me she simply can't believe it. George McMahon says, "I've never seen Stuart do anything like this before."

No one else has either, that's clear. Stuart's half-hour performance is the uncontested high point of an

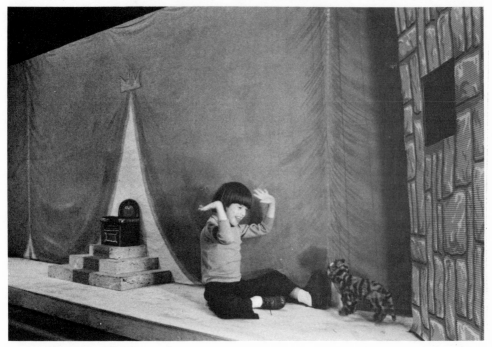

Stuart with one of the tiger cats.

afternoon that's been filled with peak experiences for all of us.

It's worth noting, in retrospect, that a whole series of occasions such as the marionnette show have occurred over the life of the project . . . and unfailingly these have been times when, if proof were ever needed, you had irrefutable evidence that the *quality* of these children's lives had not only been *improved* but filled almost to overflowing. On such occasions, of course, *everybody* was affected—teachers, administrators, arts team members, and anybody else (like us) who happened to be around.

Many of these occasions were unplanned, or at least what ultimately occurred took on a life of its own once the stimulus had been given. I think, for example, of the afternoon at Walton when Debi Ross (the team member for dance) brought over from the

Alan Short Center her group of square dancers, the Short Swingers. The group—all of them moderately retarded adults who'd been trained by Debi—performed their dance numbers in each of Walton's classroom units; but in the last one, Unit III, as Debi continued to "call" one of the square-dance figures, some of the ambulatory children moved onto the floor and began imitating the Short Swingers—and before long it seemed as though half the room had spontaneously joined in, teachers, aides, students, visitors, all of us moving happily to the spirited music.

Another instance was what the Great Oaks people referred to as their "Spontaneous Hootenanny," an occasion that grew out of the visit, one Friday morning in the spring, of a professional opera singer whose special appearances at all three project schools had been arranged by the NCAH office in Washington.

Though we were never fortunate enough to be on hand for them, it appears that Paula Mondschein's visits were memorable and impressive occasions in their own right. Afterwards, the teachers at each site were unanimous in their praise, not only for her glorious singing voice and its impact on the kids but for her extraordinary sensitivity to the needs and conditions of individual children, especially those who couldn't hear or see her. Pat Berilgen, one of the teachers of sight- and hearing-impaired children at Great Oaks, recounted the visit there this way:

Paula Mondschein was simply wonderful; we all were overwhelmed. She had our deaf-blind kids put their hands on her vocal chords and "feel" her singing; and you should have seen their expressions when they sensed the vibrations in her neck and throat. And then she did some arias—and she projected so loudly that even some of our very, very severely hearing-impaired kids heard her, I *know*.

Of the spontaneous hootenanny that grew out of this, Pat said, "Then the drama and dance people came in, and they got the feel of the situation and started dancing and singing and cutting up together, and our kids entered in—and it was just a wonderful moment." Janine Stone, the Great Oaks drama person, noted that "one of the most exciting happenings of the project so far" was the way that more and more teachers and students got spontaneously involved, singing and dancing and having fun together that morning. The experience in fact was so rewarding and broadly participatory that the arts team began to "schedule" similar happenings on a fairly regular basis, Friday mornings during the spring.

Then, too, there was the field trip the SCS kids took to the Dallas Symphony's Young People's Concert; and the informal concert that a friend of Michele Valeri's, a folksinger named Bob Devlin, staged in the woods one day on the Great Oaks grounds; and the dozen or so Great Oaks kids who took part in the parade up Pennsylvania Avenue during the National Very Special Arts Festival held in Washington, D.C., in May.

Another set of "special events" was prompted by George Latshaw's third cycle of visits to the schools. George had planned that part of these visits would be given over to puppet-making workshops for the teachers—and some wild and wonderful puppets came out of those sessions, too, plus a renewed deployment of puppet activities in the classrooms. The balance of each visit, however, was devoted to work with the arts team members on the creation of a performance of some kind which they would then "tour" to each of the classrooms for presentation to the children and the teachers. In keeping with the return of spring, these presentations in song, dance, and the visual arts were usually celebratory events on a "Search for the Sun" theme. While the visual arts team member created a living mural depicting the events as they occurred, the other artists portrayed the Sun, the Wind, the Rain, and Clouds, and George's Big Witch puppet went among the children to search for the Sun and make it shine again after Rain Clouds had covered it. Despite the planning involved in them, these collaborative performances, on what was billed as "arts extravaganza day" or a "spring arts festival" at the schools, had a spontaneous, commedia dell'arte element about them as George and the resident team trooped exuberantly from classroom to classroom for performances before the small audiences of their "special friends."

All in all, these special events which took place from time to time throughout the project seem to have produced moments that were exciting and exhilarating for the children—and greatly treasured by each school's complement of teachers and artists.

Walton Development Center, June 1979

It is June now and Roger and I have, in a sense, come full circle: we're back in Stockton, at the Walton Center, where our journey into this extraordinary world of severely and profoundly handicapped children had its beginnings last November.

This is the day of Walton's Very Special Art Festival (VSAF), the "celebration of life" that people here have been planning for weeks as the climactic—and concluding—activity of the arts project here. It also marks the official termination of the entire pilot project, since there have been similar VSAF celebrations recently at Great Oaks and SCS that have brought the projects there to a festive and colorful conclusion.

Each of these heady events has been graced by sunny weather. This, happily, has enabled the day-long series of performances, demonstrations, and participatory activities to take place—as planned—outdoors in the patios and courtyards as well as indoors in the classrooms and gymnasiums of the three schools. Each festival has been planned, developed, and organized jointly by the arts teams, the team leaders, and the school staffs. The site team coordinators—Jan Goodrich at Great Oaks, Randy

Routon at SCS, and Yvonne Soto here at Walton—
have worked closely with their respective school
administrators, Lynn Johnson, Carol Fritze, and
Ann Trujillo, on "the grand design"; together they
have planned and woven into each day's schedule a
colorful melange of arts events and activities, including many that involve groups from other schools
and institutions for the handicapped nearby.
They've seen to it that parents, other handicapped
kids, neighborhood residents, and assorted VIPs
(local and national) have been invited.

Meanwhile, the arts team members at each site
have generally been concentrating on those things
in the program that involve their own children; they
have spent the final few weeks of the project working with teachers on the preparation of all kinds of
original presentations that various groups of children are scheduled to perform before VSAF audiences on *the* big day.

Roger and I have been on hand for all of these big
days and, like the one here at Walton today, they are
truly *festive* affairs: ribbons and colored paper are
festooned everywhere; clowns and mimes (usually
drama students from nearby colleges) wander about
improvising "conversations" with you; big
compressed-air cylinders have been used to blow up
hundreds of colored balloons that people are holding;
there are sideshow activities and "special creations,"
like the series of huge cardboard packing boxes that
some Alan Short Center staff members have joined
together and filled with sights, sounds, smells, and
textures to create a multisensory environment that
the kids are taken through; rooms have been set
aside for the showing of arts/handicapped films; the
walls are filled with fascinating exhibits of the project children's artwork; drama, dance, music, and art
students from nearby universities are conducting
workshops; and there are demonstrations and skits
and readings and dramatic presentations going on
simultaneously all over the place, indoors and

out—as the crowds shift constantly, gathering at half-hour intervals to become an audience for something or other and then moving on to something else.

These VSAFs all have certain elements in common; although the casts of characters differ, the substance of what takes place is surprisingly similar. In addition to the activities noted above, each festival has its main stage for featured performers—located out of doors under a tent or on a covered makeshift stage (as at SCS and Walton) or indoors on the gymnasium stage (at Great Oaks). On the main stage, a constant round of lively (and often amplified) performances takes place before large and enthusiastic audiences: rhythm bands, jazz-rock bands (like Mike Ross's here, and the Maryland School for the Blind Rock Band at Great Oaks), singing groups, and dramatic groups (like the Denton State School Drama Class which presented *The Life and Times of Robin Hood* at the SCS festival). Another event common to all places is a wheelchair square dance (called "Wheel and Toe Do-Si-Do" at Great Oaks), an utterly beguiling configuration of kids in wheeled chairs being pushed giddily about the floor by teachers, foster grandparents, or arts team members.

The event that particularly enchants audiences at all three festivals is, of course, the half-hour performance of the Latshaw Puppets, a full-dress "puppet review" that includes amusing scenes involving many of George's favorite puppet people. Wilbur and the others perform on a custom-built puppet stage that George has designed for use when he goes on the road, a stage that can be quickly assembled and taken down but which, at the same time, enables him to work effectively behind its curtain with his big cast of characters, and the props and costumes (and voices) he's created for them. In each place, these performances are occasions of great fun, superb examples of a master artist working with humor and imagination at the craft he loves. Unfailingly, they captivate youngsters and adults alike.

Moments from the VSAFs.

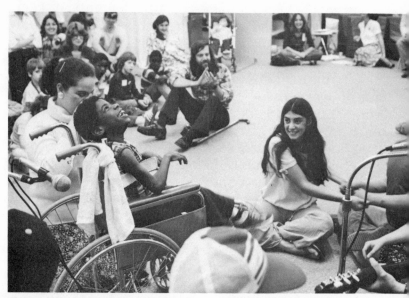

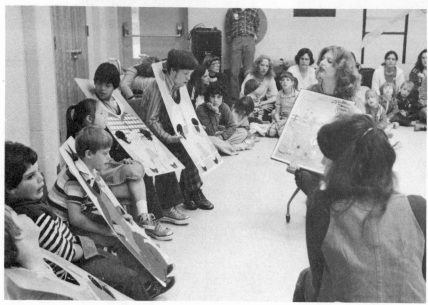

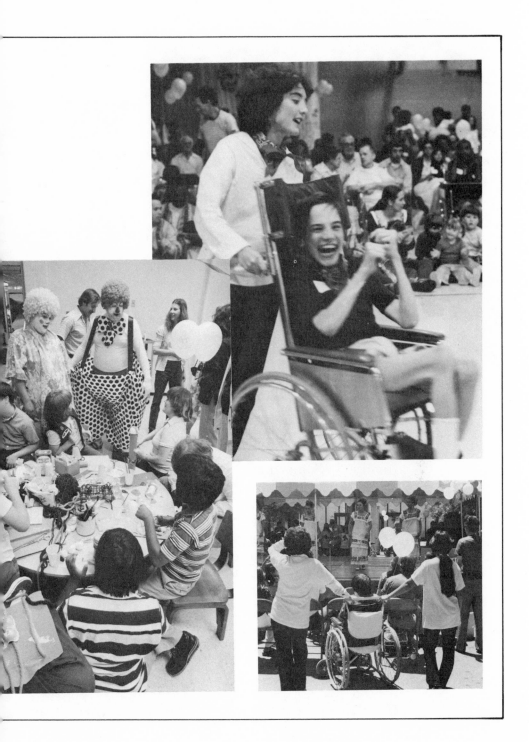

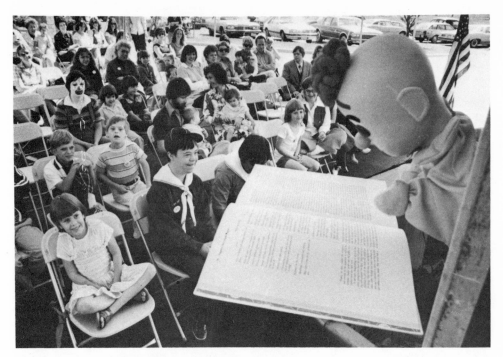

George Latshaw and his puppet people in performance.

But most endearing of all, certainly, are the festival activities in which the children themselves are involved. Sometimes they take part in the workshops the artists have scheduled, helping the artists provide visitors with a glimpse of what actually went on in class during the project; at other times you find them appearing in brief but carefully rehearsed playlets where each child has a specific action, word, and sound to contribute to the narrative, on cue from teachers or arts team members (the wolf, for example, who huffs and puffs at the little pigs' houses). They may turn up in a musical or dance presentation they've rehearsed in class with one of their teachers, or they may be found having their faces painted, clown fashion, by the team's drama person. Sometimes they'll simply be sitting together and enjoying themselves as members of the

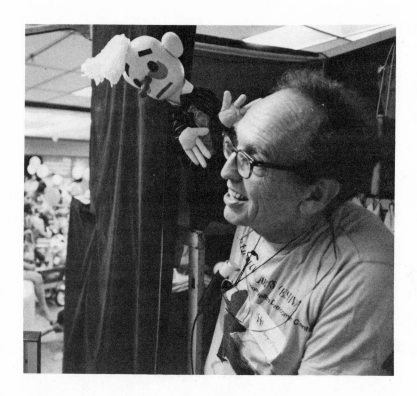

"main stage" audience. Or indeed, a very few of
the higher functioning kids may actually be taking
part in a main-stage event, performing something
they've learned painstakingly to do—as Junior did
when he led us in the "Star Spangled Banner" at the
opening ceremonies of the SCS festival; or as Guy
and Faye and several others are doing here at Walton in the square dance they've been preparing for
weeks now under Debi Ross's patient guidance.

These festivals, you realize, have several reasons for
being. You have expected that they'd be something
of an exercise in show-and-tell, a kind of demonstration of what the children may have learned during
the project, a showcase of some of the skills they've
acquired. And certainly they serve this purpose in

part: you think of the wide range of visual art on display, Guy and Faye in their square dance, the songs some of the kids have learned, the remembered responses given on cue in the playlets, and so on. But you sense that such things are not really what the festivals are all about; they are *more* than this. What they *are* about has more to do with the "quality of life" than anything else—that part of the project's goals that bear on the enrichment of these children's lives, on their social and affective development, and on providing opportunities for the same kind of peak experiences we saw revealed so poignantly in Kathy Burks's theater that early March afternoon.

In a sense the festivals are an event apart from the rest of the project; indeed, we heard a few complaints at each site to the effect that the regular work of the artists, in the classrooms, had to be curtailed several weeks early so they could help the kids and the teachers prepare their parts for the festival. At the same time, without the festivals as a culmination, the projects would all have ground slowly to a halt, and the ending would have been distinctly downbeat.

So the festivals somehow *had* to be. They served to focus people's energies and attention on a significant episode in the life of each of these three special schools. And they gave the vast majority of students a strong feeling of participating, of being a part of something special and exciting, even those who simply participated as members of an audience. Indeed for almost everyone who attended them, the festivals held a unique fascination; they were a kind of peak experience all their own . . . well worth whatever programmatic dislocations they may have created otherwise.

The arts team here at Walton has not had an easy time of it, all things considered. Two of its original members ran into difficulties after a month or so and were replaced sometime in March. Valuable as their successors ultimately proved to be, it cannot have been easy for Celeste Behnke and Maria Rubino, working in music and drama respectively, to pick up on those assignments at what was almost mid-project. Although both Celeste and Maria had some music-therapy training in their background, neither had worked previously with SPH kids and that adjustment in itself must have reduced their effectiveness somewhat at first.

Meanwhile, even Doug Genschmer (in visual arts) and Debi Ross (in dance), as the continuing members of the team, were faced with problems essentially unlike those confronting members of the other two arts teams. They stemmed mainly from the fact that Walton's teachers functioned—not in a number of small classrooms with six or less children—but in the three large teaching spaces inhabited by from thirty to forty kids each. The artists (new to this environment *and* to the children) found it difficult often to work effectively amid the distractions in this busy environment. Before long, therefore, they began conducting their arts sessions behind screened-off areas of the room, or taking the children (singly or in groups) into other rooms nearby where greater "instructional control" could be maintained. This practice was, to some extent, duplicated on occasion by artists at the other two sites but seldom to the extent employed by the Walton team members during the first several months of the project. More than anyone, perhaps, Doug Genschmer felt the necessity for this kind of isolation in his visual arts activities, which were quieter and less flamboyant than the other art forms, and required greater patience and concentration.

However, while the artists' teaching emphasis could be focused fully and more effectively on the kids under these conditions, the practice gave rise to a new problem: namely, that the teachers were being pretty well excluded from what was happen-

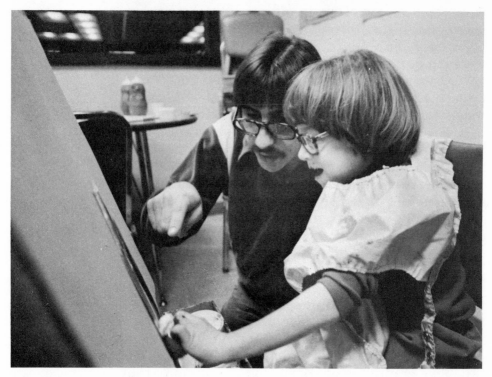

Jamie painting with Doug Genschmer.

ing during the arts sessions and were thus unable to acquire very much in the way of new teaching skills involving the arts. So, in the end, it was a practice that had to be altered, or at least modified, if there was to be any significant carry-over to the teachers of methods and techniques that had proven valuable in working with their children.

In March—at about the time that Celeste and Maria were entering the picture as the new music and drama team members—a major change in procedure was initiated at Walton. From then on, the artists remained in the units when their sessions were scheduled; they were asked to work in tandem with the teachers as much as possible, bringing arts techniques and approaches to bear on whatever the teachers were doing with the children at the time.

It seems to me the most valuable results come when the teachers guide the artists toward the IEPs, relating our activities to theirs. If a teacher has really special directions he/she wants the work to go in, the artists can be advised of this. But generally I feel it's too much for the artist to deal with. And beyond this, a concern with the IEPs may serve to constrain or restrict the artist in developing new ideas. In effect, I'm saying that I believe the artist and teacher roles should remain distinct.

Janine Stone (Drama)
Great Oaks Arts Team

Kathy Saylor, one of the head teachers in Unit II, described the situation this way:

The first month or two, each of the artists settled on a group of about six kids and they worked only with them; they'd pull them out and work with them in isolation, on some of the specific goals we'd developed for each kid. But under that approach, we—the teachers—really weren't getting much out of the artists' visits. Then, when the shift came, it meant that they'd come to *our* activities with their ideas and work *with* us when we had something going. Once we were able to share our knowledge of the kids with them, and they were able to share their knowledge of the arts, as teaching tools, with us, a whole lot of good things began to happen.

Although the changeover seems to have improved the situation for the Walton teachers, some of the arts team members (at project's end) said that they had continued to feel some frustration with this arrangement. The difficulty here appears to have its roots in the fact that they were no longer able to work systematically—in their own ways—on the individual goals of a particular group of children. And the reason that this disturbed them, one began to feel, is that they were essentially teachers themselves—and their teaching expertise happened to consist primarily of teaching the arts to *children*, not in teaching what they *knew* about this to other *teachers*. Thus they were frustrated when the em-

My feeling is that we came and worked with the obvious condition of the child and made our intuitive evaluations of his or her needs. I think we were really working on IEP objectives without knowing it a great deal of the time.

Graceanne Adamo (Dance)
Great Oaks Arts Team

phasis shifted from an exclusive effort to bring about change and improvement in the children, to one that was at least equally concerned with helping the teachers to acquire some of these change-producing skills and teaching techniques themselves.

This occurrence brings more sharply into focus a point alluded to earlier but one which became increasingly more intriguing as the project moved to a conclusion. It concerns some fundamental differences in the makeup of the three arts teams. The professional philosophy under which the members of this Walton team, and some of those at SCS, seemed to be operating was in rather sharp contrast to the core philosophy which permeated the work of the Great Oaks team. When all was said and done, in their heart of hearts the Great Oaks team members clearly saw themselves primarily as Artists (capital A) placed in a situation that required them to share their creative qualities with children and teachers. Most of those on the Walton and SCS teams, on the other hand, tended to regard themselves essentially as Teachers and/or Therapists (capital T) whose instructional tools were grounded firmly in artistic elements and approaches. For the most part, the members of the latter two teams had worked in educational settings before or were doing so presently as part of their training—and a few had even had direct experience with handicapped children. The Great Oaks team members (with the exception of Pam Lowenthal) were essentially strangers to both of these circumstances.

Knowing the IEP goals gives me a starting point and a finishing point. It saves me hours and weeks of trial-and-error experimentation, of finding out for myself the functional level of the child and what direction to go in with him. . . . Several teachers mentioned to me how pleased they were to find the arts team took time to find out the IEP goals and then to design activities to work toward achievement of those goals.

Barbara Baxley (Music)
SCS Arts Team

The basic teacher/therapist philosophy was pretty well expressed by Doug Genschmer:

I feel that if you're an artist and you think you have something special to offer, it's almost like a faith—and the only way to go about getting that across to other people is through the teaching process. You're first an artist and the satisfactions you get from your work are a vital part of your life. But then you realize there are lots of people who aren't aware of the richness the arts can bring to their lives, so it's your job to find the best way to reach them—and to me that's by teaching.

Yvonne Soto, Walton's site team leader, took this directly into the NCAH project arena by pointing out that "an artist, per se, comes into these situations saying 'here's what I have to offer' and he goes ahead and does his thing—learning from mistakes and making modifications, maybe, depending on the audience. The arts teacher/therapist, it seems to me, comes in and starts where the audience *is*—in this case, handicapped kids and their teachers. He draws on his artistry or performing background to help implement what he's teaching."

As for a description of the (capital A) Artist's philosophy, perhaps the Great Oaks drama person, Janine Stone, in a comment noted earlier, put it as succinctly as anyone:

The teachers at SCS really encouraged us to work on the children's IEPs as much as possible–although they didn't have much confidence that the objectives could be reached through dance until they saw it in operation. While I believe it's important to reinforce these objectives, the higher functioning children really need variety–so it's necessary to relax these pressures some and develop a few objectives of your own for the child, or boredom sets in. I found a blending of the teacher objectives and my own an effective way to work.

Carol Kay Harsell (Dance)
SCS Arts Team

It's not the art, it's the artist; it's not the art *form* that's essential to this kind of work, it's that you are an artist—a real artist, a capital A Artist, a special kind of person. Because a real Artist feels, senses, and looks at the world in a particular way . . . and I'm convinced that it's the kind of people we *are*, not what we *do*, that makes it work here, with these kids.

The most obvious way in which this distinction manifested itself was in the differing approaches the two camps took to the matter of working with the IEPs—the children's Individual Educational Plans. Seemingly, the Great Oaks people gave the IEPs of the kids some cursory attention early in their work but were genuinely wary of becoming inhibited by them; most (though not all) members of the other teams felt that studying the IEPs early on and becoming familiar with them gave them valuable clues about the kinds of arts activities they could begin to use with the children.

Doug Genschmer, again, spoke for most of the latter group when he said:

I'm really pro-IEP—I think that's the whole idea. If we're going to get the teachers to adopt our activities, we've got to prove to them that what we do can be fitted into the IEPs. You've got to discover the various levels of the students and then provide the activities that can best improve skills *and* let them enjoy themselves in the process.

And Graceanne Adamo's comment probably sums up the Great Oaks team's IEP stance as well as any:

What we as artists have to bring to these kids happens, I think, regardless of whatever analysis may have been made of their needs. *We* can proceed without being hog-tied by all that—so the possibilities for these kids are unlimited for us. In other words, I would hope that we, as perceptive people, could sense some needs and possibilities in them that the teachers may have overlooked, because often they're looking mainly for the more skill-oriented thing.

The elaborations on these themes were endlessly fascinating (see box on page 123). But in the end, it became meaningless to make value judgments about which approach might have been more effective, and so on, because clearly this project had not originally been structured in order to bring ultimate resolution to such matters. Inadvertently, however, its three-site design did allow these distinctions to emerge and provoke speculation.

Nevertheless, as Louise Appell had predicted, most of the good things did repeat themselves at each project site. The rewarding "Ah-hah Light" did indeed flash in much the same way in all three places. What was different was mainly a matter of attitude and style—the distinct professional attitudes each arts team took to the task at hand and the personal behavioral styles its members exhibited in action. In one group—the western contingent—one could discern more preproject study, more deliberate planning, more of a "lesson-plan" approach, more attention to stated goals; in the Maryland group, more sponteneity, more of a tendency to "wing it," more flexibility, and a great dependence on intuitive approaches.

While these distinctions in the professional orientation of the teams conditioned much that went on, the practitioners of the separate art forms seemed—on many occasions—to have a great deal in common, also. As noted earlier, much of the time you saw similar kinds of materials, instruments, and props being used, the same kinds of games, activities, and happenings being carried on, and with the same general kinds of results.

One of the more striking commonalities among the teams was the concerted effort the artists made to work with one another on joint activities, to supplement and reinforce one another's contributions. It occurred time and again, but its flowering—in all kinds of warm and wonderful ways—is exemplified by a somewhat serendipitous happening that took place late in May at Walton. What started as a drama activity in which Maria Rubino hoped to get across something about self-concept to the children had, in the end, developed into a kind of related-arts free-for-all that was tapped into by Debi Ross's dance activities and Celeste Behnke's music. As such it represents the sort of self-generating, cooperative way of working which virtually all the arts team members found to be extraordinarily exhilarating. The Walton artists do a splendid job themselves of describing what occurred, in its proper sequence:

WALTON'S ANIMAL FREE-FOR-ALL

MARIA (DRAMA): At one point I was trying to deal with the idea of self-concept and, for some of the higher functioning kids in Units II and III, I brought in some make-believe frogs . . . a big one and little teeny water frog. We worked to establish the concept of big and little, of jumping up and down, and the color green—and related them to people in the group.

Then, I brought in the live animal—a frog that was actually alive. They could touch it if they wanted, see it hop around and, because I was holding it most of the the time, it wasn't too threatening to them. I brought in a live bunny too, and he also hopped around a lot.

The week after that I came in dressed as those animals, in a frog costume first, then a bunny costume. We had worked the week before on signs for "frog" and "bunny" with those kids who couldn't speak and, when I came in in those costumes the

reaction was immediate. Little Julian gave the sign for "frog"
right away ... and when I came in as the bunny, Guy came
over and started hopping happily around. The little ones got a
bit scared at first when I came in as the frog—so I took the head
off to let them see it was me. Then I put it on them so they could
see each other in it; we'd put it on and take it off and I'd say,
"Now you're a *frog*" and "Now you're *you*," while they looked
at themselves in the mirror.

Then, the last week, I brought in makeup and some little costume things, and I made the kids up as the animals we'd been
working with. ... I had some big bunny ears and some frog
warts, and so on. This makeup activity was the *big* event for
the little ones ... they enjoyed the sensation itself, they
looked at themselves a long time and got really involved.

CELESTE (MUSIC): I knew Maria was working with frogs and I
happened to stumble onto a song about frogs. So I made some
simple finger puppets that were frogs, and then I made a log
out of construction paper, cut some holes in it, and put in some
make-believe bugs. Then all the frogs would sit on the log and,
as I sang the actions in the song, the frogs would eat the bugs
and jump in and hide in the holes.

When Maria came in one day wearing her rabbit costume, I
was in the room working on a tone-bell song (where they just
play the scale) about a little bunny that grows up. I had a stuffed rabbit at home (happily the same color as Maria's costume)
and I brought it in—and we said, "Maybe, if we play our music
well enough the bunny will really grow up and get very, very
big"—and at the climax, of course, in hopped Maria dressed in
her *big* bunny costume. So we all hopped around and sang a
song about hopping. It was quite a sight.

DEBI (DANCE): Spinning off of Maria's frog thing, I got Lisa to
jump—using a frog. I'd worked with her for weeks, but she just
wasn't getting the concept of jumping. So I got a plastic frog
and told *him* to jump down the stairs to the floor—and of
course he did. Then I gave Lisa the frog and got *her* to make
the frog jump down the stairs. Next I got Lisa and the frog to
stand on the step and I'd make the frog jump—and then I'd say,
"Okay, Lisa, *you* do it now," and she finally did it. We did the
same thing to get her to jump over a small piece of wood. We
did it over and over again—and now she doesn't need the frog
anymore.

I thought maybe it would be harder for her to associate with the frog and then transfer it to herself—rather than seeing a human do it. But she was really much more interested in the frog than a human being doing it, for some reason.

GEORGE LATSHAW: What Debi described is very close to the way I think puppets can contribute to this business, because it makes learning these things so absorbing and so interesting to the child. What she said about Lisa's having no interest in watching the human is precisely the point. Humans put so many demands on the kids that tasks like this then become very difficult to get them to do. But the puppet gives it a kind of playful feeling that's fun . . . seeing first the frog jump and then having the "frog's friend" jump . . . that's really a perfect way to get something accomplished.

And this is a perfect note—this account of some collaborative and inventive teaching—on which to end this part of the narrative concerned primarily with the project itself, with what happened when an infusion of artist-teachers took place in three SPH schools, and why.

There remains only the final attempt to assess the value of that infusion, to draw together some opinions on this from the participants, and to reflect in very personal terms on the outcomes of the project.

5

SPECULATING ON THE OUTCOMES

DOCUMENTING SOMETHING—a project, an event, or even a journey such as Roger's and mine—is one thing. You attempt to tell or show what took place as objectively as possible, but always with the knowledge that elements of the subjective and the personal cannot fail to enter in. Evaluating something, assessing what the people involved got out of the experience (whether, for example, anything of consequence was learned or accomplished), and coming to accurate and reliable conclusions about its ultimate value is usually viewed as something very different indeed.

Certainly, up until now this narrative and the pictures interwoven with it have not been strictly objective. Value judgments have surfaced from time to time. Clearly, our selection of photographs cannot be regarded as dispassionate. There have been instances where some attempt to understand a particular circumstance better—the artist-versus-teacher issue, the relative merits of small classrooms versus large teaching spaces—has led to some superficial analysis and speculation. And whether in boxed areas or in the narrative proper, the quoted comments of artists, teachers, parents, administrators, and others have pointed up the kinds of conclusions some of the project participants, at least, were coming to about its ultimate value.

And now, clearly, the reader has every right to expect that we will shift gears and provide objective, indisputable evidence that this Arts Project for Severely and Profoundly Handicapped Children and Youth can be termed a smashing success or a dismal failure, or perhaps labeled as merely "a qualified success," or possibly that its outcome was simply "too close to call" with any accuracy. Readers expecting such a cool and scientific resolution to our account will, however, be disappointed. This project was not conceived or designed to produce that kind of success-fail results—and our account is simply not susceptible to such tightly reasoned conclusions.

The twin goals of the project—to improve the "quality of life" for these youngsters through a variety of experiences in the arts and to improve their "functional skills" through the use of arts strategies—cannot, on the other hand, be ignored or dismissed out of hand now that this "first of its kind" venture has concluded its first developmental year. Has there, indeed, been discernable improvement in these youngsters along either or both of these dimensions? A reasonable question, but one the answer to which depends on a whole range of *other* questions relating to the assessment techniques used to determine it.

What behaviors will be measured? In how many children—all of them or just a representative sample? Will it be "improvement" if *any change at all* is noted? How long must a noted improvement persist to be valid? Given the extremely damaged condition of some of these children, how in fact can one determine what may or may not have been *learned*? And, short of requiring the artists to keep precise, minute-by-minute logs or having trained observers follow each artist around, *all the time*, and record his or her every move, how can we know for certain which child received how much "treatment" (of what kind) from which type of artist? We'd need that, it would seem, to know how much weight to assign *the arts* in assessing a given child's improvement—or lack of improvement? Even then, how would we know *for sure* that it had been the artist's intervention in the child's learning process which had been responsible for any changes noted? Might they not, in fact, have happened *anyway* in the course of the child's regular educational program or at the appropriate stage in his or her development?

Without resorting to complicated and expensive comparability studies—in which, say, these three groups of children (who were to participate in the arts-infusion program) would be matched as closely as possible with three other groups of similar children who would *not* be receiving "treatment" by a group of artists—these are questions about which it would be very difficult indeed to arrive at definitive answers.

An observation of Dr. Hugh McBride's—the educational psychologist from the University of the Pacific who had been asked to serve as our Project Evaluator/Data Analyst—points up the difficulty rather succinctly with respect to this particular project: "You aren't ever going to develop a standardized test," McBride says, "that works *in indisputable terms* with kids who aren't standard to start with—who are, in fact, way off at one end of the behavioral spectrum."

Nothing daunted, McBride nonetheless did proceed to gather some intriguing data about the effect of the project on these children, data having to do chiefly with the second major goal: improvement in their functional skills. To do so, he utilized two different kinds of assessment devices. One of them was an instrument he designed himself specifically for this particular SPH population, something he referred to as a "Behavioral Checklist"; it consisted of brief descriptions of forty separate actions or responses on which the children were rated—on a scale of from 1 to 5—by local volunteers whom McBride trained at each project site. This was done at four different stages in the project's life (though only three times in Dallas because the project ended earlier there). Analysis of this data would indicate whether the children, on the whole, moved up or down on the scale—on each of the forty items—during this 6-month period.

The second instrument was the Denver Developmental Screening Test, a standardized test which McBride arranged to have administered to all project children, at each site, before the project activities began and again when they were ending. "The Denver," as it's known in the testing world, has been used since the late 1960s to help professionals identify "developmental deviations" in young children from birth to 6 years of age. McBride felt it was not likely to provide us with much in the way of "indisputable" evidence of changes in the children, because of the extreme degrees of retardation and handicap that bounds their existence. But he decided to use it because it was the only standardized instrument that even came close to meeting the particular needs of this project—and, in the end, it might provide us with some findings to speculate about, at the very least.

On analyzing and reviewing the data obtained from both of these instruments, McBride found himself "amazed that we were able, in the face of generally poor rater reliability, to get the kind of data we did, though I'm not necessarily surprised that we actually saw change, per se, occurring." Without becoming enmeshed in more technical detail than I can handle, I should merely say that the results obtained from both kinds of instruments, though certainly not definitive, were positive and heartening—and leave it to Hugh McBride himself to deal with the substance more fully in the appendix.

At the same time, there is no question but that the more subjective and personal kind of data abounds. Part of this largely anecdotal evidence can be found in the random comments of project participants which have been liberally scattered throughout this account. More specifically, though, their perceptions have been drawn upon to flesh out the dozen or more

"You Get Clues From The Artists All The Time"

We're learning new things about all these kids, things we didn't really sense before. Maybe it's because we protect them so much and aren't able to change their environment very often. We just don't see things sometimes—like, I knew Jeff was funny about new people, but we never gave him the opportunity to work that through until the artists came in and starting working with him. . . .

You get clues from the artists all the time. Jeff began tracing things on the floor one day, when Pam was in here. We'd done body tracing the week before, but Jeff wasn't even involved then. But this day, he began tracing his hand—and later when I was working with him trying to get him to spell the name "Jeff" I got him started by using the tracing idea. Well—you see, I had no idea he could do that because, at the beginning of the year when we gave him some tests that have measures for telling you about tracing abilities (among other things) . . . according to those tests, Jeff wasn't even ready to begin tracing his name on paper. But, here I suddenly see that he can do it and that he found it out by himself. But I'd never have known about it unless we'd found it out through that body-tracing art activity of Pam's.

Marlene Becker
Teacher
Great Oaks Center

"case studies" of individual project children that appear in the appendix. It's worth taking a moment, here, to explain how these accounts came about and how the material in them was obtained.

By the time we came to our second round of visits to the project sites, Roger Vaughan and I had become convinced that we wouldn't be able to make very perceptive observations (photographically or

I started writing songs about the kids when I couldn't think of any more new things to do, and it went over big. Soon the teachers would ask me to do a song on this kid or that—and one day Sue came up to me and said, "I'm sorry, but little Jeffrey died before you got to write a song about him!"

Michele Valeri (Music)
Great Oaks Arts Team

narratively) about the effect the artists were having on these SPH children if we tried to keep all three hundred project kids fully in our sights. To provide a sharper focus for these observations, we decided to narrow the field down and concentrate our reporting on perhaps eight or nine children in each project school, a total of twenty-five or so in all.

We hoped to achieve a comprehensive mix, in these groups—of sex, race, kinds and severities of retardation or handicap, chronological age, and living situations. To this end, the teachers, administrators, and arts team personnel worked hard and thoughtfully with us to try to make certain that the resulting cross section adequately reflected the composition of the larger group. We made it clear, furthermore, that we weren't interested only in "poster children," nor in children whose presence in the group might smack of stacking the deck. Furthermore, we indicated that our request for such a "focused" selection did not mean that we would ignore the rest of the children—observationally speaking —from that point on; it meant only that we couldn't report intelligently on the behaviors of three hundred kids!

From within this group of about twenty-five children, we ultimately were forced—for reasons of space—to settle on twelve whose reactions and responses to the work of the three arts teams would have to stand for all the rest; they would have to carry the burden of our thesis in ways uniquely their own, and through them we would hope to reflect something of what had taken place in many, if not all, of the others.

It is interesting to note that in these twelve portraits, there are six boys and six girls whose chronological ages range from 2 to 20; their racial or ethnic composition includes seven whites, two Hispanics, one black, one Armenian, and one who is possibly Asiatic. As nearly as we could determine, the degree of handicap or retardation covered is such that three of the children fall in the profound category, six in the severe category, and three in a kind of borderline situation verging on TMR—the "trainable mentally retarded." Their causation factors include Down's syndrome, cerebral palsy, Apert's syndrome, brain damage at birth, and other unspecified problems.

To provide as much verisimilitude as possible within these portraits, a range of end-of-project comments are provided, largely by those who know the children best—their teachers, their parents or foster parents (where available), and other school staff members; on occasion the observations of some of the artists are also included.

Many of these "case study" comments were elicited during tape-recorded interviews, others from notes made on the scene, but the majority were derived from the written responses of teachers to an end-of-project questionnaire. This questionnaire asked for their perceptions of behavioral changes in the one "special focus" child for whom a given teacher had direct classroom responsibility during the project period. More specifically, it sought information about observable changes, if any, in each of the children in six broad areas: physical, affective, cognitive and social development, self-help skills, and language or communications skills; and it asked, further, whether any of these changes could be linked directly to the arts activities the child had been involved in—or whether they were changes

The nicest days here are really when we have a good laugh . . . at something one of the kids has done, or over a call from a foster parent, or when Ray stuck his head in the sliding trombone. His head's so little it could almost fit.

Kathy Saylor
Unit II teacher
Walton Center

that might reasonably have taken place anyway, due to maturation or regular classroom work.

Each of the arts team members at all three sites was also asked to respond to a questionnaire—but one that was more general in nature rather than child-specific; anecdotal comment about *any* of the "special focus" children was suggested but not demanded; thus, what appears in the way of artists' comments was generated quite randomly.

Most of the comments by parents or foster parents in these case studies were obtained in tape interviews—some conducted in midproject but the majority during the Very Special Arts Festivals at the end.

Taken together, these individual portraits evoke the strengths (and here and there the failures) of the project more tellingly perhaps than all the test data could ever do; they suggest the power the arts hold for reaching, motivating, and teaching these children—and for simply making their lives more joyous and pleasurable too. They also indicate some of the limitations as well, instances in which (as the teachers saw it) the arts processes failed to break through to, or do much for, certain kids. On these occasions, however, it becomes quite clear that the failure has been an individual one—relating to a particular child, usually one with multiple handicapping conditions—and not something fundamentally wrong with the arts processes themselves for work of this kind, not something that's inapplicable to the entire SPH population. But, in the final

You can't be childish. But you must be childlike! It's a quality George Latshaw has when he's working with his puppets around these kids.

Unidentified Artist

---

analysis, what emerges of real significance from these portraits is the multiplicity of ways in which the teachers of these children now believe that the arts can be useful to them as they go about their work.

Of the several outcomes relating to the project's "quality of life" objective, perhaps the most clear-cut and pervasive had to do with a behavioral element touched on several times during the course of this narrative—that concerned with "socialization."

It was something that happened so gradually during the six months of our association with these children that, often, I was personally unaware that a change had taken place until it was pointed out to me by the teachers or the artists. But once cued to be on the look-out for such behavioral changes, they seemed to be everywhere in evidence: in the way a kid who'd kept his head turned away six months earlier now looked you straight in the eye and smiled; in the greater ease with which teachers seemed able to generate group responses and a sense of cohesiveness in their class activities; or simply in the more relaxed and friendly ways that the children played with one another.

Not, of course, that all of these things hadn't taken place at times before the artists arrived on the scene. And certainly it cannot be said that in every instance the changes we began to notice were singularly the result of the artists' intervention. Yet the teachers themselves were more apt to mention this factor than any other single change in the children's

I'm one who believes that expectations play a great part in a child's development. If you expect little, you're going to get little.

Valerie Crivelli
Teacher
Special Care School

development—and, for the most part, they acknowledged a major role for the artists in bringing it about.

In one way or another the following comments are typical of a good many teachers' comments at all three schools.

"I'm doing my end-of-term testing now," said a teacher at Special Care School, "and the one area that I've seen the most development in is the social area. The kids have learned to be more attentive, in group activities, and they've learned to play together. Because, even if they never got any real dance concepts out of dancing (which they do), they're dancing *together*—doing a lot of things together. They're caring more about their classmates and their own friends too. Those kinds of things are what I feel the arts program has helped to take place. And that's a real gain for my kids because, before, they were into . . . well, abusing one another, or just rocking back and forth, no really positive interaction at all."

Another SCS teacher said, "I think the idea of the arts enhancing the quality of life for these kids is its strongest point. The main problem with our lower-functioning kids is that they don't know how to play by themselves. And they don't know how to relate to others, either. The arts program kinda teaches them how to sit by themselves and enjoy something, at least—listening to music, getting interested in a book, maybe, or looking at colors. They really appreciate these things on some level now."

I really thought "doing the arts" was going to be a waste of time at first, just another Big Deal that'll have us running off in all directions around here. But as time went on and things got better, you could see the progress in the kids. Now—I want every kid to be in it!

Unit III teacher aide
Walton Center

And, speaking about this at a faculty review session at Walton, a teacher said, "One thing that's struck me—and I'm not sure if the project has been entirely responsible for it, but I'm sure it's enhanced it—is that our group has learned to work better, as a group. Remember how hard we had to work last year to get the kids to stand up, hold hands and form a circle . . . things like that? Now they're getting much more used to working cooperatively together."

And at Great Oaks a teacher told me: "I found a lot of my kids learned how to handle new situations. They were getting much better about having new people coming into the room—getting used to different people. And I think that's a big socialization experience right there that the artists helped bring about."

To conclude this account on a highly personal note, I am compelled to admit that for several months at the beginning I harbored serious doubts regarding the efficacy of any so-called arts strategies for helping such children as these make any significant advances in their functional skills.

I was fully prepared to find that the quality of their lives could be enriched through a variety of arts experiences, mainly experiences in which the children were essentially being entertained and were relatively passive nonparticipants in the process. But it seemed to me that progress by a given child in the development of the more functional skills—language, fine and gross motor

After awhile you get to think of these kids as the normal kids.

Harold Rettig
Custodian
Special Care School

---

physical skills, academic and cognitive skills, self-help skills—could be just as readily achieved by good, creative early childhood teachers or therapists. Working with low-level children, especially, on such developmental matters as these—where patience, continual drilling, rote learning, and repetitive measures of all kinds were the order of the day—didn't seem to me to require the particular contributions that might be provided uniquely by artists, on an intermittent basis especially.

By midproject, however, I was finding enough instances in which it seemed to me certain artists on each team *had* been able to break through to certain children in these areas, that my preconceived notions were beginning to crumble in the face of them.

Perhaps it would be wise to insert a minor qualification here, however, something that one of the SCS teachers, Muffy Hoerner, helped to clarify for me during our final week in Dallas, when she said:

I think that maybe the arts work best on functional skills when they serve to *reinforce* a concept or an already acquired behavior, rather than really to teach it as a new idea. If, for instance, a kid is already beginning to understand about "right" and "left", putting it in a singing or a dance activity could be a really fine way to reinforce it. But I'm not convinced you can teach it from scratch that way. Or maybe the real point is, why complicate the issue by trying to make the arts do *everything*?

Another SCS teacher, Carol Epstein, probably would agree, although she put it slightly differently:

I just think that the artists brought in some new ideas in terms of teaching the old routine skills . . . things I wouldn't have thought about doing. To see how they were approaching some-

> *The arts people have gotten used to the children and the children to them—and now we've gotten used to them. We had to learn that we could* **share** *our children with them.*
>
> Unit II teacher aide
> Walton Center

thing as simple as teaching basic shapes and colors was an eye-opener—and I saw it being done in art and in music. That's what I picked up on—some new ways for getting those basic skills across.

Kathy Saylor, at Walton, took this even further when she said, "The arts seem to have a flair about them, a glamour, that I really like. I often think I use reinforcers that are kind of dull. But the arts are exciting and glamorous—and I think we should all use them a whole lot more, for skills *and* for enrichment."

Kathy Saylor, incidentally, pointed out that she felt the teachers and the artists at Walton had, in a sense, almost switched positions on the matter of skill development versus enrichment:

At first, when I thought of "enrichment" with the kids, I kinda laughed to myself. I thought, "How are the artists going to enrich them if the kids don't understand half of what's going on around them?" But I think my opinion has really changed, and the project has brought all that to life for me. I realize now that a child can go into some arts activity, participate for 5 minutes maybe, get some enjoyment from it—and leave. And it was fun and there were smiles on faces and—yes, you really *are* enriching their lives this way. It's funny: we teachers were all so goal-oriented and now I, at least, really believe enrichment is important; and the artists were pretty much enrichment-oriented and now they're really concerned with skill development, or at least challenged by it and trying to find better ways to get at it. It's great. It's a good team exchange, I think.

I find myself constantly falling back on teacher comments such as these to illustrate project outcomes—but this is probably as it should be. Certainly there was plenty of teacher uncertainty involved; uneasiness and sometimes open distress surfaced throughout the project; personality problems arose between some of the teachers and some of the artists; and there are, even now, many shadings of opinion among both these groups about the ultimate outcomes. But among the teachers especially, one finds very few who have not come to some new realizations, acquired some new teaching tools that utilize the arts or learned to apply an arts-oriented approach to their standard bag of tricks, and emerged from the whole experience with a genuine sense of discovery and renewal.

Members of both camps might like to see some changes in the ground rules next time, modifications in the structure perhaps, or in operating procedures and communications, but it would be difficult indeed to find very many people—in either camp at these three schools—who would argue with any fervor against the fundamental thesis involved here. They *know* the process works because they've either done it or seen it done. And, in the final analysis, that is the ultimate test of an idea that is at once as fragile and as powerful as this one.

Roger Vaughan and I discovered, when we had reached the end of this journey of ours, that we were reluctant to leave this now-familiar world of badly damaged children—and the people who teach them. We were no longer strangers to that environment, moving uncertainly among those who exist in it. The unknown had, to a very great extent, become known.

The children we met there can, of course, never really leave that world—not *really*, even the few who may one day be sent out to regular schools. For they take their special world with them wherever they go; they cannot ever fully escape from it.

And so it has been an exciting and rewarding experience to watch this world of theirs brighten and come alive in new ways—as artists entered on the scene and began to work (and play) imaginatively among them. This has indeed been "a first," and the artists and teachers together have done their utmost to fulfill its premise here—in the habitat of "the last of the least."

As our homeward-bound plane took off from Stockton that day in June, at the conclusion of Walton's festival, it struck me that—if the *ultimate* premise of this venture is to be fulfilled—the real journey has only just begun.

AFTERWORD

THIS ACCOUNT, readers will recall, covers only the first year's activities in what was planned as a developmental program spanning three school years. Officially termed "A Model Program to Enhance Living and Learning for Severely and Profoundly Handicapped Children and Youth," it was launched in the fall of 1978. Its planners had envisioned that, by the end of the third year, perhaps a dozen more special education facilities would have adopted this model arts program for SPH youngsters—and adapted it to their own needs and circumstances.

Despite the funding uncertainties that frequently plague almost all long-term ventures of this nature, this remarkable program did continue. Word from the National Committee, Arts for the Handicapped early in 1981 indicated that Project Years II and III ultimately did come to pass, although not to the full extent originally projected. If the program's fundamental premises were not entirely proven nor all of its expectations completely fulfilled, those two extra years appear to have sustained and focused its life-enhancing concepts and given them some much-needed growing room—and time.

Much of the information about what happened during those years comes from Marjorie Kohn, who became Director of NCAH's Arts/Project for Severely and Profoundly Handicapped as the third year began.

Two of the original sites—Special Care School and Great Oaks Center—continued their involvement with the program throughout the two succeeding years. Arrangement for continuation at Walton Development Center in California did not, in the end, work out, for a number of complicated reasons. And only three new sites were added in Year II, not the dozen or so originally envisioned.

The three new project sites were all in public schools in which at least a part of the students they served were defined as severely and profoundly handicapped.

The Carter School in Boston, Massachusetts, is a public inner-city facility providing developmental day care for students having severe and profound disabilities attributed to mental retardation. The Lexington School in Roseville, Minnesota, is a public special education school serving nine school districts in the St. Paul suburban area. The Getz School, located in Tempe, Arizona, is a public school designed to provide a developmental diagnostic educational program for children and young adults with severe learning problems.

The arts team approach, employed during the first year, seems to have been somewhat de-emphasized during Years II and III, so that, in some sites, more extensive work with local arts organizations was undertaken or greater emphasis placed on student excursions to a variety of community cultural programs. The Carter School, for example, worked with The Next Move Theatre, which sponsors a wide range of arts programs and events for the Boston schools and the city generally. At Lexington School, the principal and his staff worked closely with CLIMB, INC, a Minnesota-based artists' collaborative whose members have been active in the St. Paul and Minneapolis area schools.

In Year III, changes took place which Marjorie Kohn notes were "really an outgrowth of all that had happened the first two years." The individual sites assumed greater responsibility for the planning and implementation of arts activities. And primary emphasis was placed on developing techniques for integrating the arts with skill development.

During the year, in fact, an "Integrated Arts Activities Guide for the Severely and Profoundly Handicapped" was field tested in each site. A compilation of activities that use the arts as a vehicle to promote motor, self-care, and social awareness skills, the Guide encourages special education instructors to make adaptations of the activities to meet the needs of individual youngsters.

The Guide was developed by Kohn and she emphasizes that "it isn't a definitive set of arts activities but simply a handful of suggestions to help administrators and teachers to initiate, expand, or refine an integrative arts program in their schools. We hope it will provide a general frame of reference for a developmental and task analysis approach to learning each activity." Following completion of the field test, NCAH published that Guide in late 1981.

Bette Valenti, a professional artist and program administrator who has been associated with NCAH virtually since its inception, became The National Committee's Executive Director in 1980. Ernest Boyer, former U.S. Commissioner of Education and now President of the Carnegie Foundation for the Advancement of Teaching, presently heads the organization's 15-member Board of Directors.

Readers desiring further information about The National Committee, Arts for the Handicapped, its goals, programs, and services, can write NCAH at 1825 Connecticut Avenue, N.W., Suite 418, Washington, D.C. 20009.

APPENDIX:
SOME CASE STUDIES:
A Few
Representative Children
in Sharper Focus

ROSIE
(Special Care School)

ROSIE is a 12-year-old* who has been severely retarded since birth, when she suffered undiagnosed brain damage. She came to the Special Care School two years ago from another school for handicapped youngsters where, her parents say, she wasn't ever really happy and was never helped in ways they could discern.

Rosie is described as "friendly and personable" by her teacher, Marian (Muffy) Hoerner, who adds: "In a lot of ways, Rosie is a typical 12-year-old in that she likes to experiment with makeup, plays 'mommy' by dressing up, and can spend hours at her desk writing her name." Rosie has no expressive language, but her receptive language is excellent and she is now learning sign language to help in her communications skills.— JE

MUFFY HOERNER
(At Project's End):
Rosie doesn't get frustrated quite so easily now. She's more willing to try new experiences and, in fact, is becoming quite a little "ham." ... She's not as shy with strangers as she was in January —and I think the fact that the arts team was constantly present-ing her with new faces, and people who were nice, made her more comfortable with strangers. Due to the regular group activities offered by the arts program, she also seems to interact with her peers more now.

Rosie has always "babbled" in the past, usually when she was especially happy or when she was with her parent—but she babbles *more* now, and we've noticed a definite increase in this during dance class. . . . She's definitely more willing to participate in activities of any kind, and all the arts programs, we think, contributed to this factor. . . . Rosie's physical development per se has changed little; however, she's considerably more willing to try harder—that is, she'll mimic a physical movement much more quickly than she did in January. We think that this would most likely have occurred at *some* point, but not as soon. While all the arts activities helped in this—in the sense that she was involved in things where she could make use of her limited physical abilities and feel good— the dance program was the one Rosie enjoyed, and particiapted in, the most.

*In the Case Studies included here, the initial statements describe the children as they were during the first project year, 1978–79.

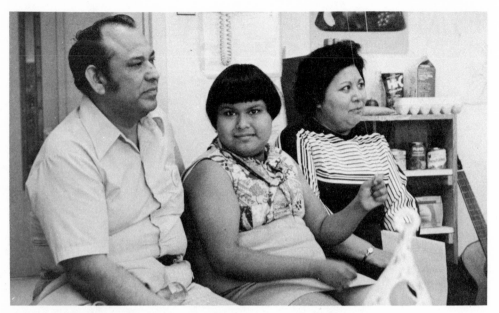

Rosie with her parents.

ROSIE'S PARENTS
(In May):

Rosie's definitely been making a lot of progress since the arts program has been going on. She's begun to do things for herself—she's more independent [this, despite Muffy Hoerner's observation that she seems to have remained fairly constant in this respect. — JE]
Lots of times, in the morning before we're up, she'll fix her own cereal. And we see her put on her clothes, wash dishes, or vacuum the house (she likes to get the dust off)—but a short while back, she never did any of these things.

She tries to communicate with us a little bit more too. She never actually said much of anything, ever before; but she never really *tried* to communicate as much as she does now, either. She uses a lot of sign language—we don't know all of the signs ourselves, but we can usually tell what she's trying to say to us.

All in all, Rosie seems to be much happier now. We think it's happened because of the fine way the school has worked with her since she came here. But really these past few months seem to have increased it more—made it all happen faster!

*

[It should be noted that Muffy Hoerner did not think that Rosie's cognitive development nor her self-help skills were influenced visibly by any of the arts activities.— JE]

ELMER
(Great Oaks Center)

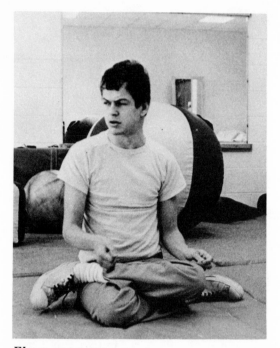

Elmer. (Photo by Molly A. Roberts)

ELMER is an earnest, slightly-built youth whose chronological age is 20. He's a member of Marlene Becker's class in room 124 at Great Oaks Center, a class of older students who have, for the most part, been diagnosed as profoundly retarded and who require modified behavior management techniques. It has already been pointed out (see pages 33–35) that Elmer functions at *different* age-levels across a group of five or six development characteristics—from a 2½-year-old level in language development, for example, to a 4½-year-old level with respect to gross motor skills (see also pages 76 and 77 for other references to Elmer).

On the behavioral scale used at Great Oaks to assess student behavior and develop objectives to meet individual priority needs, it has been noted that Elmer has two outstanding areas of difficulty—rebellious behavior and stereotyped behavior. The latter reflects his rather constant tendency to hunch forward on his chair and rock back and forth, and his habit, when left alone, of playing ceaselessly with strings or repeatedly waving his arms. His rebellious streak comes out in his rather frequent stubbornness, his failure to attend consistently to assigned tasks, and his habit of "running away" from situations that give him difficulty.

His teachers indicate that, most of the time, Elmer will participate in classroom activities to some degree and will follow directions on simple, unsequenced tasks. He seeks attention from adults often, they say, but will on occasion attempt to "interact with his peers." Some of the goals and objectives that Marlene had developed for Elmer this year included "encouraging peer interactions through group games" and "improving his attention to fine motor skills by increasing the amount of verbal praise."— JE

MARLENE BECKER
(At Mid-project, In March):
He's more independent—they *all* are, really, in this class. We're learning things about Elmer that we didn't really know before— like beating out a rhythm, and experimenting with Graceanne's spiral-cloth Snake. This kind of creativity was something I'd never had a chance to see before. But I've known Elmer so long I could see he was ... well, coming out of himself during the arts activities, because the artists were picking up on his excitement about things and his enjoyment of different activities.... When you have a class with behavioral and emotional problems, such as we work with here, you *know* there's intelligence that's locked up and really hard to reach—but we get in a rut and it's hard to break out of that; you set up a routine and you stick to it. The arts approaches give you a chance to break out of it and discover a lot of good ideas that can liven up that routine when you're back in it. When the artist and the teacher are working on these things together, as we've done with Elmer and the others in this class, I can watch what's going on and say, "Hey, he *knows* this"—or "He really *can* do that" and I can pick up on that in my own work later on. It's so great because it's giving me all these ideas and giving me inspiration as a teacher—and I guess maybe I've given the artists some ideas they can work on as well, because I've seen *them* pick up on things *I* do.

MARLENE
(At Project's End, In June)
It seems to me that Elmer has been performing to his maximum potential in all areas in response to the artists and their activities. For one thing, his cognitive development showed improvement—he learned a sequence of events (pasting blocks together) and remembered that sequence from week to week. As much as we've worked on pasting things to-

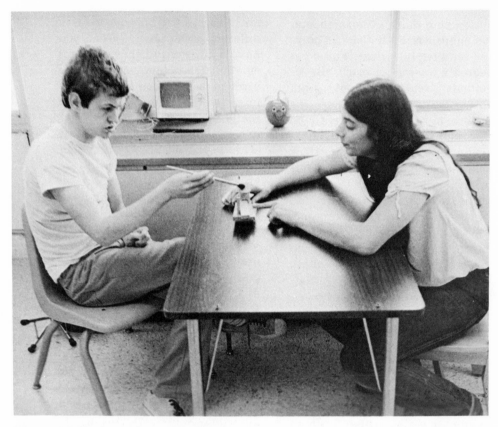

Elmer with Marlene. (Photo by Molly A. Roberts)

gether, we *never* got that result until the arts team came. He could always do each step after a demonstration—but this year he learned to complete the whole task without a demonstration!

Elmer used to have difficulty in showing affection for others; the problem is, when he likes someone he can get overly attached, refusing to part with that person. When that person is in the room, he would insist on sitting next to

him/her [see Pam Lowenthal's comment, page 76]. He'd become very stubborn when not allowed to do this—but now he may pout a little but he no longer stubbornly refuses to move. Also, he began volunteering to participate in the artist's activities. His response was greater during these activities, he showed interest in a wider range of activities, and his level of participation was greater. In other words, the arts were very "motivating" for him—they spurred him to function to the best of his abilities.

His physical development has remained pretty stable. The arts people certainly gave him more opportunities to *use* his abilities —to crawl, dance, manipulate— but he didn't learn too much that was new, except that he can now follow a rhythm by beating a drum. I think he could probably do this before, but we were not aware of it; we discovered it through the arts team.

His communications skills have definitely shown improvement: he's putting two words together without prompting now, and he's "signing" his name and *my* name. He's signing more often independently and appropriately in class—and the arts people helped by encouraging him to use a variety of signs in different kinds of situations. . . . We specifically worked with sign-language skills during music time. Music seems to be very reinforcing for Elmer, so having him sign along to the songs was an excellent motivator —and I'm sure it helped him practice putting several words together. This then carried over into other situations since he'd become used to "speaking" in longer sentences: we signed "blue shoes" to "Blue Suede Shoes" and "lion sleeps" to "The Lion Sleeps Tonight."

Elmer's social development has always been fairly high. Even so, it was a pleasure to see him interacting with the arts team people, and getting true enjoyment from their visits. He not only volunteered for activities, but he used all or most of his abilities to complete them successfully.

Maybe I could end with a clue of another kind: normally, during the day, Elmer usually runs to the bathroom frequently. But when the artists were here, he never even *asked* to go!

All in all, I guess only self-help skills seemed to be entirely unaffected by any of the arts activities.

REGINA
(Walton Development Center)

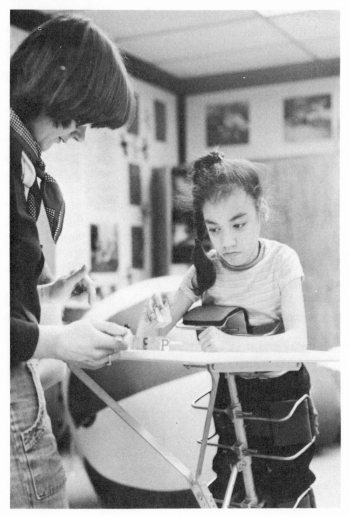

Regina with Kathy Saylor.

"SHE'S A beautiful girl, and she's smart," says her teacher, Kathy Saylor, of Regina—adding, "of course, she's one of my favorites. She's the type of person who, for many years, people thought couldn't do anything. And then we turn around one day and she's crawling—a few feet and then flopping down on her stomach at first—but she's crawling" [see box, page 30].

Regina was born prematurely and her parents noticed at about 3 or 4 months of age that "she seemed not to be making any progress." At about 1 year and 3 months of age, she was referred to the Delayed Development Unit at Walton, where she was enrolled. At that time, it was noted that "Regina is a severely handicapped child with cerebral palsy, has a marked hearing loss, and has a very slow development." She did not roll over until she was 2 years of age and, at 3, she was able "to sit alone with poor balance or even no balance."

In due time she was admitted to the regular Walton classrooms and now, at 11 years of age, she is assigned to Unit II. Her teachers note that while she's not toilet trained, she's a self-feeder, and is very aware of surrounding activities; she is able to use her hands to manipulate objects and can put rings on a stick. She signs for "eat" and "drink" and manipulates her wheelchair effectively around the unit; she has leg and joint problems, though, and she's placed on the prone stander quite a bit to keep for joints flexible. — JE

KATHY SAYLOR
(At Project's End, In June)

Regina truly enjoyed participating in the project; she isn't a very social child but she always attended when she was being enter- tained. . . . She has become more aggressive lately—for instance, she reaches for and attempts to manipulate the limbs of others to get them to do things for her. I regard this as a positive change; it may have been nurtured a bit by stimulating her interest in the exciting and fun things that the artists were providing, as opposed to self-stimulatory behaviors. . . . She's become more independent, too, in terms of using her hands to touch, explore, and manipulate stimulating instruments.

Regina's communication is through signing, of course, since she is severely hearing impaired. Any advances in signing have been as a result of food rewards, . . . however, she definitely has an interest in sound production. She recently acquired a hearing aid and this, along with much exposure to sounds (a variety of pitches and tones during participation in arts project activities), has increased her "tolerance" of a group situation under these limited circumstances. Her interest has been kept as long as 30 minutes, which is quite unusual for her.

This responsiveness to or awareness of external stimuli is an area where I've noticed a change that could be connected with Regina's participation in the project. She's clever enough to hide her awareness of staff and regular activities; however, when interesting sound makers are carried into the room or a team member comes in dressed in an elaborate costume, she seems engrossed in them. I think perhaps the key here is novelty. Regina is quite naturally interested in new or fresh things in her life.

DOUG GENSCHMER
(Visual Arts Team Member):

Regina (or Maria) in Unit II were often left alone with paints, a brush, and paper—and I'd come back and see the look of joyful accomplishment when they'd successfully applied paint to paper. . . . well, *that* was affective development as far as I'm concerned. Also, for a girl who normally responds to food rewards, Regina was able to do some painting for a short time without the material going to her mouth.

CELESTE BEHNKE
(Music Team Member):

I found that Regina was able to lengthen her attention span in music—and indeed she enjoyed *every* music activity I brought in. She would find a way, no matter

what, so she could experience the sounds and the music being made. In fact, I was most impressed with the response of almost all the deaf children—Wendy, Jason, and Regina. They were very open and responsive!

MARIA RUBINO
(Drama Team Member):

During face painting, Regina had some unique responses. When I did her face the first time, she just looked in the mirror and rubbed her face (to see if it would come off?). She then put her head back to let me paint more. She would smile and laugh when the grease paint glided over her face—and if I stopped she would pull my hand toward her face for more. She also looked at herself a very long time in the mirror.

*

[Kathy Saylor commented that the arts activities did not seem to have any particular effect on Regina's physical and cognitive development, nor on her self-help skills.— JE]

LORI
(Special Care School)

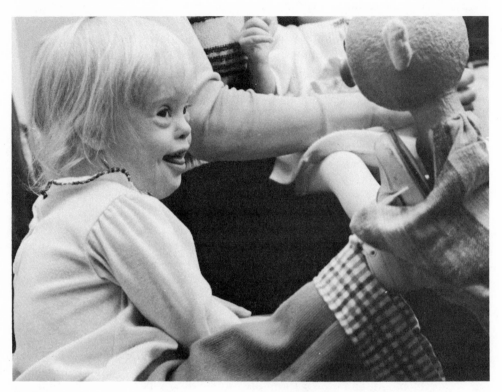

Lori.

DOWN'S SYNDROME IS the term presently applied to children who used to be described as "mongoloid." They are afflicted with a genetic disease characterized by an irregular number of chromosomes. In addition to their severe retardation, Down's syndrome children have rather a stereotypical appearance: light, silky, or very fine hair, somewhat slanted eyes, and no whorl or pattern to their fingerprints. Their foreheads seem to predominate because their hairlines are very far back.

Lori, a blonde and blue-eyed 2-year-old in the Infant Stimulation Class at the Special Care School, is a lovely and almost classic example of a Down's syndrome child. In the opinion of her teacher, Valerie Crivelli, Lori has great potential because her parents started her in a Mother/Infant Program when she was very young. It's said that Down's syndrome children who receive stimulation very early in life and are prodded constantly toward further development can progress to higher functioning levels much more rapidly than those who don't begin such treatment until they're 3 years old, and of school age.

Nonetheless Valerie believes that Lori will have some kind of disability all her life. She'll always be functioning behind her chronological age; she'll never be completely independent and will always need some kind of care. "People used to believe," says Valerie, "that anyone who had mongolism, as they called it then, would be severely retarded all their lives, but that may not hold true today. So it's difficult to predict at this point how far Lori can ultimately go, how much she can achieve."

Presently Lori functions on an 11-month level in gross motor development and is on a 15-month cognitive level. She's beginning to stack blocks, says a few words (bye-bye, Mommy and Daddy, etc.), and can point to simple body parts and facial features.

Lori's parents (her father's a school principal and her mother's a school nurse) are members of a local Down's syndrome parents association which advocates reducing the age of the public school program from 3 years to birth. Lori was their third and last child, and there is apparently excellent rapport within the family

for and about Lori—as much as possible she's treated as a normal member of the family.— JE

VALERIE CRIVELLI
(At Project's End, In June):
Lori is able to play independently and is now "brave" enough to stand in the center of the room with no assistance. She began school as a very quiet, inactive child. This *hardly* describes her now. She is very active, seeks out peer interaction, vocalizes and babbles appropriately and frequently, . . . and the arts program has helped, I believe, in changing this profile. It has given Lori many opportunities to express herself through music, art, and puppetry.

She's able now to do simple puzzles, can discriminate between several common objects, and can point to familiar objects in a book. The use of puppets and the visual arts has helped in bringing about these cognitive gains—especially in the area of body parts. She can point to body parts now with almost 100 percent accuracy.

She's also more able to cope with group situations; she's now willing to wait her turn and she's become much more active and cooperative in active play. The art activities especially contributed to this since they called upon her to function in a group setting—and she had to participate in order to receive praise and rewards. She shows more of an interest in her peers and is now imitating gross (large) movements as well as some fine movements. So, the arts program has certainly helped her social development.

Lori has become much more vocal, too; her babbling is sounding more and more speechlike; she's able to say several words—and more are emerging. All of these speech developments relied heavily on the use of puppets to get imitation of speech patterns and vocal play.

Finally, in the area of affective development, Lori has made great strides. She's now beginning to give the puppets emotion and to talk to them. She plays well with her classmates and shows a definite interest in their feelings. Again, this area has been directly affected by the arts program—the puppets particularly.

TIM MORRIS,
Recreation Specialist:
Lori does seem to be more independent! The arts may have helped her to feel better about herself—and this, in turn, seems to have helped her come out of her shell. . . . She seems to be trying to walk more, and is becoming more involved in "ball" activities, things I think would have occurred anyway due to maturation—but I think the arts, and especially the dance program, did help to stimulate it. . . . I defi-

nitely believe the puppets helped stimulate Lori's language skills. She has really become quite a "babbler," and this is probably due to her acquaintance with all the puppets.

ALLISON CROCKER,
Speech Therapist:
I feel, from what I've observed of Lori this year, that she has learned how to respond and be comfortable in many difficult situations and with many different people. This certainly was aided by the arts experiences this year at school. . . . She's more verbal, too, though I think her receptive language has increased more than her expressive skills. But the puppets certainly helped—she would play pat-a-cake and wave bye-bye to the puppets constantly; in fact, she was extraresponsive with the puppets—showed a lot of affection, hugging and cuddling them more when she played with them. . . . Lori has become much more outgoing during the course of the year, and I think all the attention of the arts people aided this greatly.

*

[Valerie, and the others as well, noted that neither Lori's physical development nor her self-help skills seemed to be particularly affected by the arts program.— JE]

ANTONIO ("WUMSIE")
(Great Oaks Center)

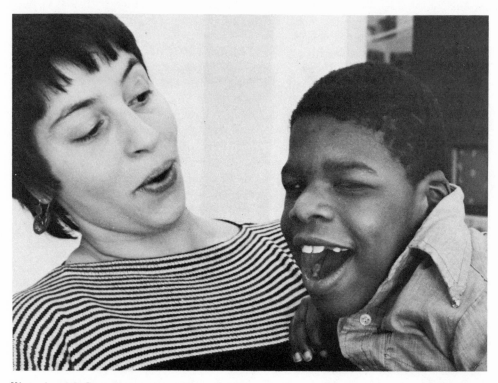

Wumsie with Graceanne.

IN A GOOD MANY instances, it is not possible to determine the precise cause of a child's mental retardation—and the file, in such cases, simply reads "etiology unknown."

This is the situation with Antonio, a 9-year-old boy who was admitted to Great Oaks when he was 2½ years of age and has been there ever since. His diagnosis at the time read "mental retardation of unknown etiology, spastic quadriplegia and impaired vision." He is nonambulatory but his teacher, Sima Breiterman, reports that "he has good head control, establishes good eye contact, and can move along the floor on his back by pushing or rotating his body with his feet."

He startles easily—and this often leads to a seizure with mild but visible tremors. Sima also noted that he is "receptive to others . . . . usually smiles and/or laughs when held, played with, or spoken to."

Antonio, who has somehow acquired the affectionate nickname of "Wumsie," must still be assessed using the Infant Learning Accomplishment Profile. His most recent assessment, in September of 1978, indicated that he does not function above the 7-month level on any of the developmental scales.— JE

SIMA BREITERMAN
(At Project's End, In June):
This past year, overall, Wumsie's progress can best be described as "blossoming." He is more active, more responsive, more interested, and more sociable than previously. I suspect that maturation may be the main contributing factor in all this—but certainly *all* the experiences he's exposed to influence his maturation and development, and the arts project was another experience in Wumsie's life that must have influenced his "blossoming" in some ways.

For example, during the past year, he's demonstrated some progress in the area of physical development—he's more active, appears to seek out independent movements about the classroom more often, and has initiated more of an intentional reach for objects within his environment. Through involvement with the arts activities, and during dance especially, he was moved around, held, and played with—activities he obviously enjoyed—and these movements most likely helped to facilitate some further gross motor development.

Wumsie has become more responsive to social interactions; he's more aware of them—and he's responding positively to affection. When approached to be picked up, for example, he begins smiling and laughing and showing excitement. While his increased responsiveness is most likely due to maturation and more opportunities for varied experiences, perhaps the number of arts team people passing through Wumsie's life has contributed to these developments.

I don't really feel, however, that the arts played any role in terms of Wumsie's self-help skills, his cognitive development, nor his general independence.

ADRIAN

(Walton Development Center)

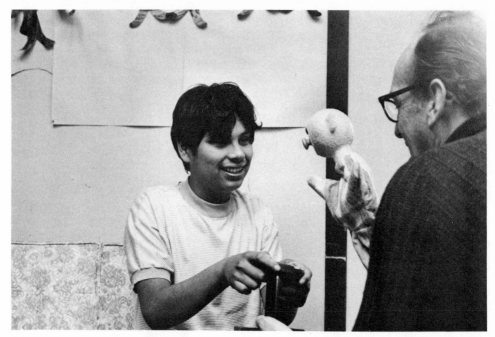

Adrian.

ADRIAN, whom we soon began referring to as "Old 44" for the faded football jersey he invariably wore, is the youngest of seven children. His father and mother are residents of Stockton and Adrian lives at home.

He's an amiable, curious, and intensely sociable 16-year-old whose face never fails to break into the warmest, most beguiling grin whenever anyone catches his eye. Rosie Jiminez, one of his teachers in Walton's Unit III, notes that his retardation stems from what she refers to as "chronic organic brain syn-

drome," resulting from oxygen deprivation at the time of his birth.

Adrian didn't talk until he was 4 years old, but he is, today, regarded as relatively high functioning, somewhere within the severe category. He walks, rides a bike, and swims; he can sort objects, imitate simple conversations, understand simple concepts, and make a few picture identifications. His teachers say he enjoys music and loves to dance.

Among the goals established for Adrian this year are such things as stringing beads, threading his belt through the loops, folding construction paper after a demonstration, and pointing to body parts on command.— JE

MARILYN BUNUG, A Unit III Teacher (At Project's End):

I came into Walton halfway through the project, but it seems to me that Adrian seems to enjoy life more now than when I arrived. It is one thing to say Adrian's behavior is better, and his motivation level higher, but to see him bubbling over with joy as well as being aware and involved is a beautiful sight. At these moments he is experiencing life to the fullest—and this means much more to me than whether he can sit quietly in his seat and obediently perform his task of putting pegs in a pegboard, say.

He's a lot more open and expressive of his feelings (both positively *and* negatively!), more aware of other people's feelings —and caring about them (he tries to help others and is concerned when kids cry or misbehave).

I do feel that some of this can indeed be attributed to the arts project, especially the music and the drama activities. The warmth and intimacy that was established in the one-to-one relationship between these arts team members and Adrian was beautiful. These people accepted Adrian in his uniqueness and worked with him with respect and care . . . and he felt this and responded. I feel this has carried over into his being able to understand and like himself more, and also to trust and care for other people.

He uses language a lot more to express feelings, in problem solving and social exchanges. His receptive language skills have also improved—he's not only taking in data but integrating information. In the cognitive realm, he's much more focused on what he's doing, and his motivation for accomplishment is stronger. He's also more cooperative and self-initiating—more aware of other's feelings and needs; he'll *help* you with something in addition to simply cooperating with you. He wants that positive social interaction. He feels freer to express himself, is less frustrated, and trusts others more. In general, he's exhibiting more acceptable behavior and depending less on aggressive ways in which to get that social interchange.

All this, as I mentioned earlier, seems to be founded on that warmth and spontaneity with which the arts team members approached him; it was literally a "joy producer" regardless of the activity being emphasized any particular day.

In terms of self-help skills, his eating habits have improved and maybe even *that* could be credited to the arts team, because he cares more about pleasing those adults he likes now. The only thing that seems unaffected by the arts program is his physical development, I guess.

STUART
(Special Care School)

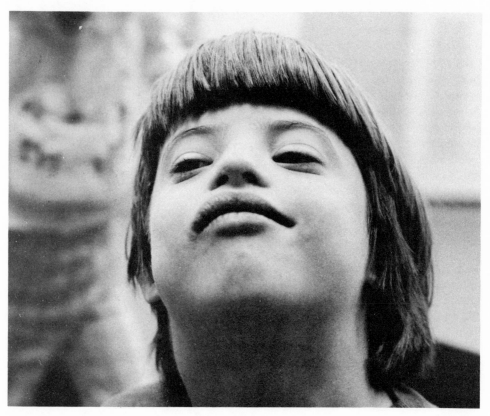

Stuart.

STUART was diagnosed as a Down's syndrome child at birth. There were no infant programs available in the area at that time so it wan't until one was established at Special Care School around 1972—when Stuart was 2½—that his parents enrolled him at SCS. "That isn't really late," says Joan Tyner, his teacher," except that *now* we have kids coming to us when they're still infants—and the stimulation they get from such early intervention seems to make a real difference."

Stuart is now 9 years old and is "on the border between severe and profound," says Joan. "You can't call him profound because he's walking, but he has some physical handicaps as well."

Apparently Stuart has very definite likes and dislikes: he likes language group activities, music, and puppet play, his teachers say; he dislikes playground-type activities, with the exception of the swings. His communicative abilities are limited to the vocalization of syllables and the use of gestures. He can walk independently, roll, and throw a ball.

He is described as very affectionate toward adults once he gets to know them fairly well. His teachers say that he learns best if something is made a part of his daily routine. At the same time, he frequently gets overly involved in sensory activities: he likes to touch and to *feel* the puppets, for example, but often he will simply use a puppet for self-stimulation purposes—to bang it against his teeth, his ear, or his head.— JE

JOAN TYNER
(At Project's End, In May):
The arts seemed to me to have an effect on Stuart in every area except his self-help skills. Probably, though, the area in which they helped him the most was in his affective behavior. He's begun to show more affection to adults, he wants to be held more, he laughs more, and he makes more verbalizations. For another thing, he adjusted well to the different kinds and numbers of people who worked with him; toward the end, he'd walk over and sit down in the "music area" the minute he saw Barbara come into the room. This kind of exposure has helped his

social interaction too. And he's simply become more generally *aware* of his peers, of adults, and of his environment.

I guess he's responded the most to music and to the puppets. Bringing puppets into more activities with him has increased both his expressive vocalizations and his receptive language. By learning to give the puppets an action of some kind, he's begun to reduce his self-stimulating behavior with them a good deal, too. And I think the puppets, music, and the other arts have helped him become more independent.

The dance program seemed to reinforce Stuart's walking and coordination and give him an opportunity to practice balance and increase muscle strength. Some of these physical skills were going to develop with or without the arts program; however, the program provided him with increased opportunities for doing all these things, challenging and motivating him. For example, the trip to Kathy Burks's puppet show gave him a chance (and much motivation) to climb the stairs to the stage to get at the puppets and play with them. His performance up there with those puppets that day was something special; none of us could really believe it.

And finally, I guess, Stuart has begun to explore objects in his environment more—especially those that make noise. He seems to be willing to initiate moving *toward* objects, such as the swings, the

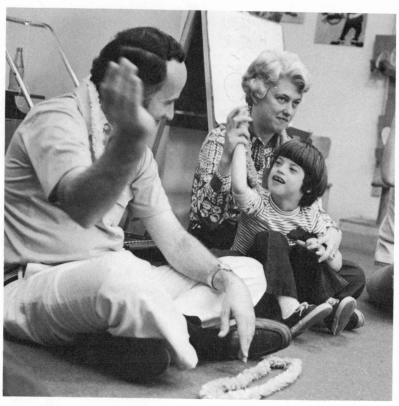

Stuart with his parents.

slide, a rocking horse, the autoharp, and the piano. And I think the arts program made a difference in these things too.

STUART'S PARENTS
(At the VSAF In May):
Stuart is more aware of things going on around him now, in general. He's more alert, a great deal more curious, and more independent. He's doing more exploring around the house—a whole lot more, just this spring.

Let's put it this way: he's been out here for seven years and, up to now, these things have never happened. So I guess you could say that the arts program here this spring has *reinforced* these developments—at the very least. Maybe he was ready for it, but it certainly has flowered this spring, that's for sure.

When we're driving in the car, he's always paid attention to certain landmarks, but now he's apt to lean forward, look out, and pay attention to things and not just sit there absorbed in himself.

He's not talking at all—but he's responding, and he's initiating things he never did before. He's making more demands now, and he keeps on being quite persistent about it too. But the main thing is he's more *aware*—and more curious. He brings us things to identify. At home, he's constantly asking questions (either by signing or using body language) about what's on the stove or the table—he looks in all the pots, wants to know what's in them, and he explores and manipulates all the things on the table tops. We think he's always had *the ability* to do these things, but he's never had the desire or the motivation to do them before.

He's always enjoyed playing on the piano at home, but he's getting to know the difference now between banging and something that's really a repetition of the same note. There has always been a real rhythm to it, but now it's getting ... well, I guess you might call it "creative." He's doing it more carefully with his fingers—not just banging away monotonously.

Raising Stuart is really just like raising a normal child except that he goes through his developments at a slower rate than other kids—the same patterns, the same sequences, but just taking much longer. Half the time we don't even think of him as being different from his two older brothers. Actually it's really helped them; they're both concerned about him, and we never have any problems getting them to babysit.

The main thing, in raising a child like Stuart, is that you just have to be more cautious and watchful all the time—and that's especially true now that he's beginning to get more curious and aware ... so he doesn't hurt himself.

HOLLY
(Great Oaks Center)

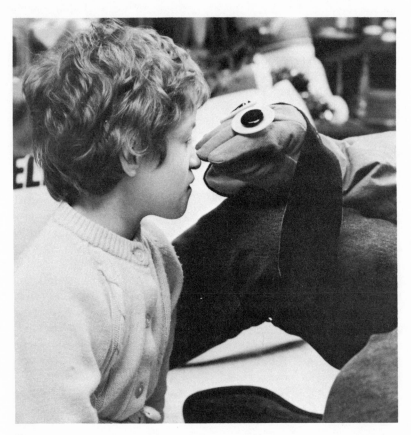

Holly.

As HER TEACHER, Angie Blatchley, points out (page 47), Holly is a little 10-year-old institutionalized child who likes to tackle challenging tasks but who's also stubborn and snobbish if she doesn't think those tasks are interesting or worth her while. (Like most of us, perhaps.)

Holly suffers from some sight loss, and she has a hearing loss in her left ear that fluctuates between moderate and severe. She has some physical handicaps as well—deformities of her hands, etc.—and she's been diagnosed as severely retarded. According to her most recent Assessment

Summary, conducted in September of 1978, she functions in most developmental areas at levels between 1 and 2 years.

She's unable to function independently in most of the usual self-help categories, is easily distractible yet can (when she wants to) attend to various skill activities for up to 3-minute time spans, independently. She can come to a standing position, stand, and walk *only* if someone is supporting her. She has trouble climbing stairs, even with help—possibly due to her problems with depth perception.

Holly is able, nonetheless, to do successfully such things as place rings on a stacker, put chips in a sorter, pop beads together if her hands are held steady, and—with assistance—screw together plastic nuts and bolts. She's at the prewriting stage of scribbling, but she will independently pick up a crayon or magic marker and scribble (in circles) on a paper. She understands and responds to several verbal commands ("stand up," "come here," "eat," "pottie," and "look," among others) when they are accompanied by the appropriate environmental cues/situations. She expresses anger by crying, grunting, shaking her head, or moving away from "undesirable" persons or activities.

The Assessment Summary concludes: "Holly is very alert and curious this year, and all her programs will be designed to encourage her to "think" about what she has to do. . . . Time each day will be given to experimental ideas and activities to determine her thinking abilities and encourage spontaneous participation in new activities on her part. She appears more willing to participate in familiar, slightly novel situations—and this year, as many such novel situations as possible shall be implemented."

The arts program appears to have come along at precisely the right time to provide a vast array of new situations and activities to test Holly's abilities in these "slightly novel" if *un*familiar ways.— JE

ANGIE BLATCHLEY
(At Project's End):
Generally speaking, Holly has made definite progress in many developmental areas this last year. She's benefitted from all the input she's received and has learned to sort out and better generalize from incoming stimuli. She's still apprehensive in new situations but is more willing to participate in unfamiliar activites with unfamiliar persons. The arts project was indeed one of the many major input systems that have helped Holly this year.

In the cognitive realm, Holly has learned to solve simple problems (i.e., how to get out of an undesirable position). I don't think the arts people had enough time with her to really work on problem solving, but I would think they could have developed excellent ideas for this area if they'd had more time.

Because she becomes frustrated easily, she's had to learn to cope better with her feelings during the arts project. She was especially frustrated during the art activities ... because (except for the finger-painting–with–food activity) she didn't enjoy them and there wasn't enough reinforcement in them ... she often had a tantrum or threw down the materials. This, however, is a necessary part of learning how to cope!

Holly is used to having positive interactions from adults around her. . . . She wants to please them but she also wants to get a lot of praise for any of her efforts. She's rather selective in responding to new persons, therefore—that is, she really appears to like new people who go out of their way to like her. So it was interesting to watch how she reacted to (and with) the personalities of the various arts people. . . . She took immediately to the dance person and willingly responded to her constant encouragement. . . . She was positive but a little frightened of George and the puppets, but definitely interested. . . . Her reaction to the music person was fascinating! She didn't dote on Holly, didn't push—but waited for Holly to make the first move— and Holly did! That was exceptional because, for once, no one hugged her first. She had to demonstrate interest to get some

feedback. An excellent experience for Holly!

Holly's language/communications skills are still puzzling to me ... because she doesn't appear to understand *language* itself but, rather, gets situational cues from her environment. It's helped her, therefore, to be around new faces like the artists' and try to decipher what is going on in unfamiliar situations ... to watch her environment more closely, and put things together to make sense of it all.

One major goal for Holly this year was to become more tolerant of and less upset with new activities, people, and environments. This she has done—and well. She was most interested in the dance activities as they involved swinging, prancing, twirling, and marching—she appeared to enjoy them all.

Finally, Holly has made major gains in the area of physical development. She is more readily "cruising" along furniture and coming to a standing position while holding on to furniture for support. . . . She's also standing independently away from a wall for approximately 2 to 3 seconds, which is a major achievement. Even though she's still fearful of independent walking, she has made efforts to try many of these *preliminary* activities and, I hope, with intensive training she *will* begin to walk in the near future.

Have the arts programs played a part in this? Well—one can

never say precisely why a child has learned new skills. Perhaps Holly would have been "ready" for them regardless of the program input. I am personally delighted when my kids learn new skills, no matter why or how. So, to me, her intensive exposure to the various art forms and personalities provided this year seemed to be another way for her to adjust to and experiment with her environment.

GRACEANNE ADAMO
(Dance Team Member):
Holly has trouble accepting new demands made upon her—such as being moved in a certain way or executing a particular new developmental skill. I tried to make a multimedia happening a part of every nonambulatory class, where all adults in the room sing and march supporting, carrying, or wheeling the children around the room. One day, I put Holly in a wooden classroom chair *backwards* so that she would feel secure and be able to hold on—and then I pushed her around to the music. It seemed to work!

FAYE

(Walton Development Center)

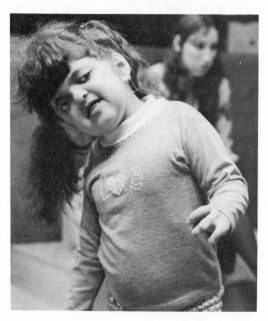

Faye.

ANOTHER DISEASE, far less common than Down's syndrome, which can strike children at birth and has a genetic basis is called "Aperts syndrome" (or disease). What are referred to as "multiple congenital anomalies" produce severe retardation and a number of unique physical malformities: misshapen head, bulging eyes, and webbed fingers and toes—that is, all digets on both the hands and the feet are fused.

This is what has happened to Faye, a 9-year-old girl in the Walton Center's Unit I who was placed with foster families in the Stockton area soon after her birth. She now lives with several other Walton children in the home of Mrs. Iris Colvin, an elderly woman who is listed as Faye's foster mother.

Pat Schmidt, Unit I's head teacher, made the comment to us in March that "quite truthfully, the improvement you may see in Faye and some of the others here is not necessarily due to us, her teachers, or to the arts people; it's because of the good foster homes, and I'd like to see them get some credit. If you think Faye's good here, she's probably even more fantastic when she's at home with Mrs. Colvin."

Faye's degree of handicap places her somewhere in the severe level of retardation. She had surgery several years ago to separate her thumbs from her fingers and give her a more functional use of her hands. She doesn't talk yet, but she can see and hear, and her teachers say she does quite well with everything, considering. In fact, she's regarded as something of a "ham" around the Unit.

Pat Schmidt continued: "The thing we like about Faye is that we've known her for a long time now—and when we got her she was very, very small and didn't do much of anything but stand and walk painfully. She was very withdrawn . . . didn't want any physical contact . . . and wouldn't eat anything but cottage cheese and bananas. All of this was partly the result of not being in a good foster home. Her parents withdraw her from that one though, and put her with Mrs. Colvin—and that's made a fantastic difference."— JE

KATHLEEN BOWMAN AND DOLORES LEWIS,
(Unit I Teachers, In June):
We don't see any changes in Faye's self-help skills, in her language development, or in her cognitive development that could be traced to anything in the arts program particularly. She's always been an independent child; she's also very well coordinated and has always been able to keep time to music in a rhythmic motion; she's continued to express herself by humming and whistling—as she's always done.

Faye isn't the type of child to hold hands—she likes to initiate interaction on her own terms. She's never been very good at following directions in any type of activity associated with physical contact. So we definitely feel Faye's attitude has changed by being involved in the folk dancing which encouraged her to interact with others on a physical level. Not only did she participate willingly but—from the expressions on her face—she seemed to genuinely enjoy the dancing. She smiled through that entire performance during the VSAF.

We're not sure how willingly Faye *cooperated* in the beginning, during all of Debi's square-dancing practice sessions; all we have to judge by is Faye's willingness to go with Debi when she came in to get her each time for rehearsals. And something else — in terms of social development — is that, before, she'd only allow physical contact with those of us on the immediate staff—and that was with reluctance sometimes. But now, here was Faye allowing a total stranger to hold hands with her.

And finally, she now seems to be more sensory-oriented, and it seems to have stemmed from her participation in finger painting, coloring, clay, and water-play activities, things she was reluctant to participate in before.

AURORA KNOLD, Special Education Assistant, Unit I (After The Very Special Arts Festival in June):
We were all just amazed to see Faye up there on the stage doing the square dancing. She never did it before, and we never in the world thought she *could* do it. We stood there with our mouths open: here was our Faye-Faye doing a little dance up there. She doesn't want anybody to touch her (except us because we know her well), and to see her touching people during the dance was amazing—and then coming out and curtseying at the end! Frankly, I think now she could balance on one of her fingers if you asked her to!

JONELLE
(Walton Development Center)

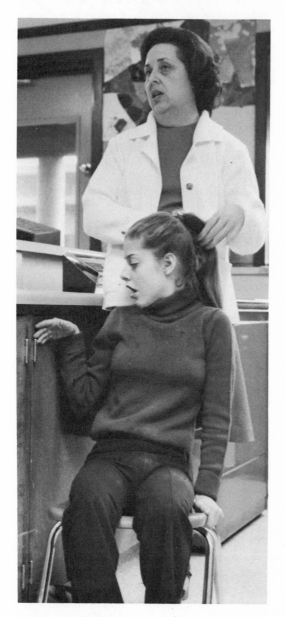

Jonelle and her mother.

JONELLE IS a remote, starkly pretty girl of 16 who's in the Walton Center's Unit III. Her retardation and her physical handicaps are the result of severe oxygen deprivation at birth; according to her mother, the deprivation lasted 8 minutes, a full 3 minutes past the point when permanent, irreparable brain damage occurs.

She lives at home with her parents who are both very caring people; an older sister has married and now lives elsewhere, and an older son is away at college (see box, page 166, for more details on Jonelle and her family).

According to her Unit III teacher, Pat Handel, Jonelle is toilet trained and has few accidents, walks but is very unsteady, has no speech but does make sounds and once in awhile will smile, laugh, or clap her hands. She shows some awareness of certain adults (smiling faintly and reaching for them) but shows little awareness of other children in the Unit. "I've observed her crying only once," says Pat, "and then I couldn't determine the reason."

She has "grand mal" seizures and takes medication to control them. Her mother believes that she becomes particularly seizure-prone when she's hyperactive. The seizures never last beyond

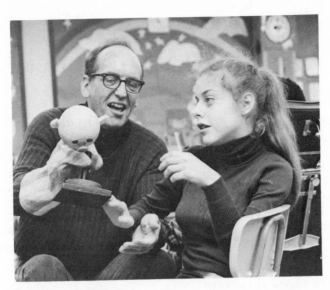

Jonelle with George.

half an hour — and often she will recover from them in a very few minutes

She's on a low functioning level, her teachers say, perhaps because it's difficult to motivate her to do things. She sits staring, often with her head turned to one side, and seems to have no real interest in anything. There is a grace and composure to her at these moments that is most arresting. "I think," her mother says, "that if she were a normal child, she'd have a disposition that's very warm and affectionate."— JE

PAT HANDEL, Unit I Teacher (At Project's End):

I haven't been able to observe any change in Jonelle's physical and cognitive development, nor in her self-help and communications skills.

Affectively, however, Jonelle has shown an increase of affection toward others over the past few months. She used to be very selective about showing affection (mainly to me and her family). But I've noticed that she responded more to the arts team than to regular staff members— and I've been enthusiastic about her change. When this display of affection occurs, I've encouraged others to respond to her in the same ways. This new, more affectionate behavior in Jonelle also involves her social development, of course, but she still doesn't socialize with other children.

I'm afraid this is about all I can point to where the arts seem to have played any role—but, then, no *other* changes (*period*) seem to have taken place in Jonelle during this time.

"Why Don't You Put Jonelle In An Institution?"

Jonelle was born in November of 1963. I have since heard that there were more retarded children born in the mid-1960s because of an experimental program the medical profession was involved in at that time. This program involved simply massaging a newborn child's chest rather than spanking to shock them into crying. And that's exactly what the doctor did with Jonelle.

Jonie's situation was brought on entirely by lack of oxygen at birth; if they have more than 5 minutes' lack of oxygen, then there's permanent, irreparable brain damage. She was deprived for 8 minutes!

At about 2 months I noticed she wasn't responding to sounds—and she didn't smile, or coo or gurgle or anything. So I kept taking her to doctors and questioning them, and they'd say they could find nothing wrong. Finally I said to one of them, "Look, Doctor, she's *not* sitting up, she's *not* crawling, she's *not* trying to stand—something's got to be wrong!" And ultimately, of course, she was diagnosed as retarded.

My other daughter's lived in constant fear that one of her children would turn out like this—and I've just told her that this is one of those things that could happen to anybody, anywhere, regardless of profession, education, race, anything.

I've been criticized, by relatives even, who say, "Why don't you put her in an institution? You're depriving your other children of so many things." And I just feel *this* way: there's so little I can plan to give Jonelle—I can't give her an education; I can't ever plan to give her music or something like that. I can't ever give her a wedding—all those things. What else *can* I give her besides love? As long as I'm physically able, I will keep her at home with us. I'm not blind to the fact that the time may come when I won't be able to any longer. But I'm not going to institutionalize her until I have to. I just hope she doesn't live to be too old—I hope I'm able to outlive her.

Jonelle's Mother
(at Walton Development Center)

JIMMY
(Special Care School)

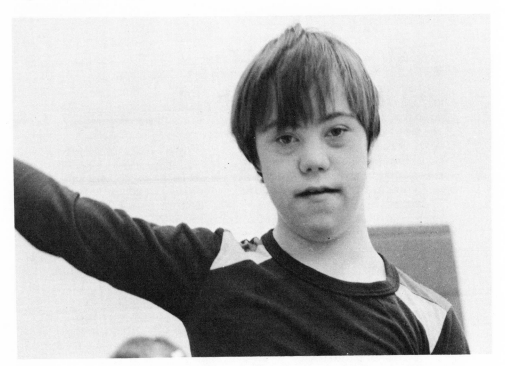

Jimmy.

JIMMY IS a relatively high functioning Down's syndrome child, who's in Alice Blume's Intermediate I class at Special Care School. He's 13-years old, ambulatory, and although he often appears somewhat passive and shy, he has what his teachers describe as a "very pleasant, happy, and 'ready-to-please' attitude toward his classmates and his teachers." They add that he enjoys group activities, especially when they involve some form of art or music.

Academically and socially, Jimmy is functioning on about the 4½- to 5-year-old level; his fine motor development, however, is on about 2½-year-old level. He has good visual memory and has learned to read and sign fifteen different survival words. He has a large vocabulary, although he often speaks in very soft tones—almost whispers—and his sentences usually consist of only two or three words. He knows and can write his name, his address, and his phone number.

"When You Have A Retarded Child . . ."

I was 45 years old when Jimmy was born—and let's put it this way: statistics tells you that the later in a woman's life the birth, the greater chance there is for Down's syndrome to appear in the child.

What difference has Jimmy made in our lives? How do you describe it? Who knows what it would have been? Dear me—we were too old to raise a baby to begin with—we had two daughters, 13 and 16, at the time . . . but both of them are much finer young women than I think they might have been otherwise. One's a teacher, the other's a nurse, and they're both very empathetic, very responsive and caring people. They might not have picked those things up along the way, not in today's world.

So he's given us great enjoyment, but at the same time there's a fantastic lot of pain. There's always a good deal of pain raising children anyway—but it's a different type with Jimmy.

We continually do more and different things than our comtemporaries. Our social life is entirely different because to get a sitter is very difficult—now the girls are up and out. . . . We took him camping; he almost grew up around a campfire, in a playpen far enough back so it wouldn't bother him. . . . We didn't have the parties at the house that the girls would ordinarily have had—we couldn't plan slumber parties because he was ill a great deal of the time and that might just be one of the nights we were sitting up all night with him.

We learned very early that the photographer's favorite seated portraits of Jimmy were for the trash basket—a photograph is such a bare naked thing, really. But the snapshots that caught him *responding* to something, they really showed *our child*, where a posed portrait would have been a completely blank statement.

And through long years of practice, you become a very adept worrier. Even now, I can't put him out to play with the children across the street because he's still not dependable crossing the street. So the watching is constant—and the supervision.

When you have a retarded child, it's as though you'd been stripped naked. All your personal pictures of yourself—as a young girl, a college girl, a young woman, a wife, and mother—your pride, your self-image, your pretenses and rationalizings, they're all stripped away—completely gone—when you have a child like this. I've found this to be true of nearly all parents of retarded children. No one's ever *completely* honest, of course, but I truthfully don't believe there's any need any more for my husband and me to *impress* other people. You go through life for awhile, always putting your guard up. And suddenly you've had it! There's absolutely nothing you need to guard against any more.

Jimmy's mother
(at Special Care School)

Jimmy has fairly well developed self-help skills; he's completely toilet trained and bathes himself with little assistance. He's just about mastered the art of tying his own shoes. (See box, pages 168-169 for general comments by Jimmy's mother.)— JE

ALICE BLUME, His Teacher, and DEBORAH BARTSCH, Teacher Aid (At Project's End, In May):
Probably the main art form that's had an impact on Jimmy is dance. It's made him more of an aggressive person, in the best sense of that word. Before, he was pretty shy—though he's always been an affectionate, happy child, he tended to play by himself; he wouldn't touch or talk to people—or even look at you much. Now, though, he's begun to talk in a much louder tone of voice. He walks up to other people in the classroom and starts talking with them—and he initiates much of this himself, without prompting. He'll grab a ball from somebody and run, sometimes—and he'll walk by a classroom, look in, and say "Hi" to the teacher there.

Maybe it wasn't all the dance—but he really does love to dance. And the dance classes with Carol Kay and Rosie have provided . . . an appropriate setting for him to express himself through creative movement. He's always been a very limber and well-coordinated boy but, before this, he tended to get into dance activities at inappropriate times in the classroom, and his movements weren't focused or controlled.

In both dance and art, Jimmy was either given materials or allowed to make music in whatever ways he wanted to—and this seems to have helped him become more independent.

And the dance and music activities seem to have reinforced many things Jimmy'd begun to learn in the cognitive realm, such as survival signs, time concepts, and response-type concepts.

His overall aggressiveness—his outgoing qualities—are a positive step forward for Jimmy, though, because of his earlier tendencies toward much more passive, inward-oriented social skills.

JIMMY'S MOTHER (At The VSAF In May):
I think all the children seem to be enjoying life so much more. They're stimulated to greater activities. And with Jimmy—why, it's spread to all his activities . . . his relations with other people, especially. The increase in his vocabulary alone is fantastic—and the way he speaks up. And he has such a good time dancing now. He's always liked dancing, but he does seem to be enjoying it more now.

I really do believe the arts have played a part in all Jimmy's developments this spring . . . because he's really had the worst winter imaginable in terms of his health. Every viral infection that came along, he got it first—and then the rest of the school got it. But he's still had a wonderful year and so much has happened to him that's positive and good!

DARLENE SEGUIN
(Visual Arts Team Member):

The visual arts activities allowed the kids an avenue of expression that didn't necessarily require verbalization but in many instances acted as a catalyst for conversation—and this was very much the case with Jimmy.

Jimmy needed conversational stimulus and, through particular visual arts activities (finger painting and balloon puppets, for instance), this was accomplished. From muffled whispers that had to be prompted in the beginning, Jimmy was soon speaking spontaneously during art in clear, audible phrases. This so impressed his teacher that she incorporated the balloon-puppet to stimulate his speech in class.

BARBARA BAXLEY
(A Music Team Member):

There are a number of instances I could cite in which music was used to improve the children's functional skills. . . . Jimmy, for example, in Intermediate I, began to talk out loud more consistently as a result of participation in group music sessions—and certainly by playing the part of the duck in the skit for the VSAF, "The Little White Duck," which Kathy Burks and I worked out.

ROSIE GONZALES
(A Dance Team Member):

I don't know whether this ever had any effect on Jimmy or not, but one day I took him out on the parking lot and I said, "Jimmy—you and I are going to shout out our names as loud as ever we can!" So I'd shout out my name and then ask him to shout out his. I can't say that he ever shouted as loud as I did, or as loud as he might be capable of shouting, but he sure didn't whisper it any more after a few tries.

JIMMY'S MOTHER IN MARCH:

In terms of communication, he doesn't have to have a puppet in his hand to make-believe. He'll use his hands alone and have separate entities doing things. For instance—he'd been watching the old Mickey Mouse show, and the phrase they use to end the program and begin it had the words "because we *like* you" in it, and they fascinated him. He'd try to say "because," but all that would come out would be gibberish—like "gubicabish" or some such. Then, one day, we were riding in the car and those hands of his began going—and one hand said (through Jimmy, of course) "gubicabish" and the other hand said sternly, "No—it's *because!*" That hand said it perfectly, and it was telling the other hand how to say it. So he doesn't always need the puppets to play make-believe and come out with some very revealing things! His hands are his puppets.

CHUCKY AND HIS CLASSMATES

(Great Oaks Center)

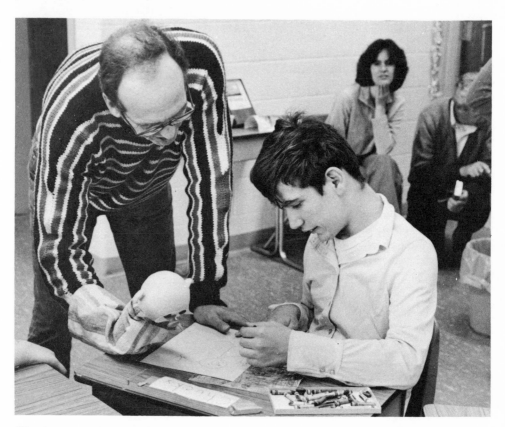

Chucky.

IN ROOM 120 at Great Oaks there are seven students, six boys and one girl, all in late adolescence and ranging from high profound to moderate (or borderline trainable) in their functioning levels.

Charles (or Chucky, as everyone calls him) is one of them. He is a 15-year-old listed as "borderline" who is among those selected for "special focus" at Great Oaks.

To give a bit more verisimilitude to these cases— and because the teachers in Room 120 (Phyllis Jones and the teacher's aide, Ada Smith) reported in considerable detail on the effect of the arts program on all but one of Chucky's classmates—this particular case study will include those comments, as well as a closer look at Chucky himself.

Chucky, at 15, is one of the youngest students in the room; there is also an 18-year-old, two 20-year-olds, and two 21-year-olds.

Chucky has no apparent physical handicaps. Yet, despite his high functioning level and his good classroom behavior, he can't be admitted to the public school system because he has difficulty riding on buses with large groups of people—either the large school-size buses or the smaller green buses used on the Great Oaks grounds. Something in this situation is distressing to Chucky, leading to disruptive and aggressive behavior. A program of gradual "bus-orientation activities" has been undertaken by the school to help Chucky overcome this difficulty so he can attend school in a less restrictive environment.

Otherwise he's among the highest functioning youngsters included in our group of "special focus" kids. Chucky's tests reveal that he likes books and magazines, can talk about pictures, and can read a few words; he listens attentively to long stories and can repeat them back to you; he can write letters and copy words, write the numbers 1 to 50 from memory, count to 100 with reasonable success, tell time to the hour and half-hour, tell the days of the week and the date, and give the correct year. He has very good eye-motor coordination. He's shown an increasing interest in his appearance over the past year, and is able independently to groom himself in front of a mirror.

The only thing preventing him from leaving the Great Oaks environment and continuing his schooling elsewhere is Chucky's bus-riding behavior; this also presents problems with field trips at Great Oaks as well. It is behavior he began the year displaying in the classroom as well—biting, kicking, shouting, and hitting others when he became upset or there was a change in the daily routine; but his overall classroom behavior has shown much improvement over the year, his teachers say, and there has been *some* progress in his bus-riding behavior—but not enough.— JE

PHYLLIS JONES, *Chucky's Teacher, and ADA SMITH, a Teacher Aide (At Project's End, In June):*
Essentially, while the changes in Chucky were not due entirely to the arts team, in our opinion, there have been changes in his behavior due to the overall flow of

people in and out of the classroom this year, and this includes the arts team members.

At the beginning of the project, Chucky didn't like following directions for activities initiated by new people. He'd show his usual agitation when someone new came into the room and interrupted the routine. Toward the end of the project, however, he would accept these people coming in and was willing to cooperate with them. (His coordination, movement, and gross motor skills were very good; he's just a little stiff yet when he's dancing.)

When people enter the room now, he greets them appropriately, usually tells them how much he loves them, and will shake hands or hug people.

When the arts people started coming, it only took him a few sessions to overcome his new-person frustrations, enter into the routine, and follow directions. He seemed to feel less comfortable with drama than with the music, art, and dance, but he soon began looking forward to all their visit.

On Scott:
[age 20 and listed in the profound category]
Scott gained alot from the arts people coming in. He likes to watch for awhile and then participate when he wants to. When the project first started, he showed increased aggressive behavior both during and im-

mediately following the music and dance sessions. And he wouldn't participate in the visual arts session at all the first couple of meetings. Soon he began cooperating more, however—toward the end of the project his aggressive, self-abusive behaviors decreased, and he started to join in and cooperate—and ended by enjoying the sessions.

On Terry:
[age 21 and also listed as profound]
Terry seemed to have gained the most from the arts project. He usually communicates in sign language even though he's capable of talking; he has a slight hearing problem so he often chooses to speak in a whisper. He never sang in the regular music classes with the teacher from the Center, but by the fourth month with the arts team, Terry was involved in the music sessions to the point of singing as well as playing the musical instruments. Beyond this, however, when we'd practice routines or complete projects *after* the sessions with arts people, Terry would speak loudly and was always most helping during these follow-up activities.

On Jon:
[age 18 and listed as moderate]
Jon had a lot of problems prior to the project that hindered him from really getting involved in the sessions when they started in

January. By April, though, Jon was a great asset to the sessions—and especially the music, where he sang loudly and acted like a true member of a rock group. He took his visual arts activities very seriously: when he was coloring his body tracing, he made certain it was "perfect"; he'd color for awhile and then stand aside looking at it to see what he needed (or wanted) to add.

On Karen:

[age 15 and also listed as moderate]

Karen doesn't like it when unfamiliar people give her commands. So she too was rather uncooperative during the first couple of music sessions. She'd act as though she hadn't heard the directions or would turn away from the instructor. At the end, though, she was ready to try almost any new idea the arts people offered, and carry out directions they'd give her without hesitation.

On Chucky R.:

[age 20 and listed as profound]

Chucky R. also gained a great deal from the experiences with the arts people. He began very soon listening to directions more, and following them. At first, he'd grab objects without asking and refuse to let someone else have them. At the end, though, he'd wait until his own turn came—and always gave the objects back at the end of the sessions. He really looked forward to the arts people coming in and enjoyed being involved in the groups.

Overall, our feeling is that the arts project did a good deal for all the kids in our room, in one way or another. We're sorry to see it coming to an end.

PROJECT EVALUATION —A SUMMARY

THE FOLLOWING is a summary of an evaluation of "A Model Program of Arts to Enchance Living and Learning for Severely and Profoundly Handicapped Children and Youth." The evaluation was conducted by Hugh J. McBride, Ph.D., Evaluation Consultant/ Data Analyst, University of the Pacific, School of Education. A copy of Dr. McBride's full report is available upon request from Thomas H. Quinn, Professional and Reference Book Division, McGraw-Hill Book Company, 1221 Avenue of the Americas, New York, NY 10020.

The purpose of the first year of this project was to implement a model program in the Arts for Severely and Profoundly Handicapped Children and Youth. The project design would: (a) improve the quality of life for these individuals, and (b) improve their functional skills through the use of art strategies.

The evaluation objectives of this first year of the project are:

1. Assess the impact of the model on the quality of life for severely and profoundly handicapped children and youth and the functional skills of these individuals.
2. Evaluate and document the results of the model program through statistical data analysis.

METHODOLOGY
The Denver Development Screening Test, a standardized screening device, was chosen as one of the evaluation instruments. The other instrument, called the Behavior Checklist, was developed specifically for this project.

Description of the Instruments

The Denver Developmental Screening Test (DDST) is a screening device designed to sort out those children who have a high probability of being developmentally impaired.

The criteria for selection of the DDST were:

1. Standardized format for the administration and a standardization established on 1,036 normal children to determine at what ages they could do each of the items.
2. Ease of administration—DDST can be administered by parents, teachers, or paraprofessionals, with minimal training.
3. Inexpensive test kit.
4. Time of administration.

In addition to these criteria, the DDST addresses four areas which are inherent parts of the Functional Skills objective of the project:

1. Personal/Social—that is, tasks which indicate the child's ability to get along with people and take care of himself.
2. Fine Motor Adaptive—that is, the child's ability to see and use his hands to pick up objects and to draw.
3. Language—that is, the child's ability to hear, to understand, and use language.
4. Gross Motor—the child's ability to sit, walk, and jump.

The test form is made up of 105 tasks written in the range of accomplishments of children in the age range of 0 to 6 years.

The Behavior Checklist was developed in order to provide a record of behaviors that might increase or change in some way during the implementation of this project. Dr. McBride, through consultation with staff at the three sites, developed a list of dependent variables.

The following are examples of these dependent variables: attention to sound-preference, attention-span with objects, body-control preference, vocal control-preference, observation of environment, image recognition, facial affect, eye contact, hyperactivity, property-abuse, participation during activities, and completion of activities.

177

The instrument was field tested at each site. Information from each of the centers was again collected, analyzed, and synthesized, and a final version of the items was generated. An instrument was developed containing 40 items and five levels of development along a continuum for each items.

Denver Developmental Screening Test
Statistically significant change occurred on 25 items on the DDST. The data indicated the magnitude of the change was in a positive direction, that is, from "Fail to Pass".

Behavior Checklist
The Behavior Checklist was administered around the fifth of each month from January thru May at the Great Oaks Center in Maryland and the Walton Development Center in Stockton, California. It was administered on the fifth day of every month from January thru April at the Special Care School in Dallas, Texas. The Dallas Center did not participate in data collection in May because of conflicts with the May 5th Very Special Arts Festival. This event served as the culminating experience of the project at each center. Special Care School held their festival earlier as their school year ends before that of the other two centers.

Data on each child was recorded monthly on Scan Tron forms. They were then collected by the art team leader and forwarded to the Evaluation Consultant/Data Analyst. Each behavioral item was coded and punched on IBM cards along with required demographic data. A program format using SPSS Statistical Programs for the Social Sciences was utilized to analyze the data.

Initial examinations of the data from the three centers revealed that the distributions of scores was markedly skewed, with extreme measurements at one side of the distribution. A decision was made to use the median as the measure of central tendency.

Table I shows numbers of medians which increased each month by center.

NUMBER OF ITEM MEDIANS THAT INCREASED BY MONTH*

DATES	DALLAS	GREAT OAKS	WALTON
January–February	22	27	17
February–March	26	21	29
March–April	22	12	22
April–May	—	29	30

*By chance, one would expect 20 increases each period.

SUMMARY

Data analysis of the first year of this project indicates that behavior change consistent with the project's objectives did indeed occur.

Statistically significant increases in 25 of 105 items on the Denver Development Screening tests indicate gains in the opportunity for improvement in the quality of life for these children through the arts. *That this improvement is reflected on an instrument which provides for few gradations in skill levels is also impressive.*

Positive changes were noted on 23 items per month on the 40-item Behavior Checklist. Improvements which related directly to increased functional skill levels, which are prerequisite to improve quality of life, were noted.

Implications: It is speculated that this improvement relates to the novel experiences provided by the project. The willingness to introduce new and exciting activities was an inherent feature of the art teams' orientation toward the children. The children tried new things, became more physically invested in their world, and consequently improved in the skills measured by the item.

Since no control group was utilized, these changes may be attributable to maturation or other learning experiences. The mean age of the children in this population was 11 years; in all likelihood they had been in school programs for at least six years prior to the project. We might conclude that even in the presence of earlier intervention this change did not occur. However, it was not until this project began that movement of this magnitude occurred on these developmentally low-level skills.

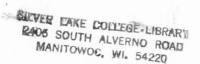